Drugging Our Children

Drugging Our Children

How Profiteers Are Pushing Antipsychotics on Our Youngest, and What We Can Do to Stop It

SHARNA OLFMAN AND
BRENT DEAN ROBBINS, EDITORS

Childhood in America
Sharna Olfman, Series Editor

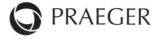 PRAEGER

AN IMPRINT OF ABC-CLIO, LLC
Santa Barbara, California • Denver, Colorado • Oxford, England

Library of Congress Cataloging-in-Publication Data

Drugging our children : how profiteers are pushing antipsychotics on our youngest, and what we can do to stop it / Sharna Olfman and Brent Dean Robbins, editors.
    p. cm. — (Childhood in America)
  Includes bibliographical references and index.
  ISBN 978-0-313-39683-0 (hardcopy : alk. paper) — ISBN 978-0-313-39684-7 (ebook)
1. Pediatric psychopharmacology.   2. Adolescent psychopharmacology.   3. Child mental health.   4. Antipsychotic drugs.   I. Olfman, Sharna.   II. Robbins, Brent Dean.
  RJ504.7.D76   2012
  618.92'8918—dc23   2011050591

ISBN: 978-0-313-39683-0
EISBN: 978-0-313-39684-7

16   15   14   13   12   1   2   3   4   5

This book is also available on the World Wide Web as an eBook.

Visit www.abc-clio.com for details.

Praeger
An Imprint of ABC-CLIO, LLC

ABC-CLIO, LLC
130 Cremona Drive, P.O. Box 1911
Santa Barbara, California 93116-1911

This book is printed on acid-free paper ∞

Manufactured in the United States of America

Medical disclaimer: This book discusses treatments (including types of medication and mental health therapies), diagnostic tests for various symptoms and mental health disorders, and organizations. The authors have made every effort to present accurate and up-to-date information. However, the information in this book is not intended to recommend or endorse particular treatments or organizations, or substitute for the care or medical advice of a qualified health professional, or used to alter any medical therapy without a medical doctor's advice. Specific situations may require specific therapeutic approaches not included in this book. For those reasons, we recommend that readers follow the advice of qualified health care professionals directly involved in their care. Readers who suspect they may have specific medical problems should consult a physician about any suggestions made in this book.

Contents

PART II. DRUGGING OUR CHILDREN: ETHICAL AND LEGAL CONSIDERATIONS

PART III. DRUGGING OUR CHILDREN: SOLUTIONS

Acknowledgments

I wish to thank my coeditor Brent Robbins and all of the authors for their thought-provoking and original chapters, which are based on years of research, advocacy, and clinical work that has improved quality of life for countless children. Special thanks to my son, Adam, who kept my computer humming and my software up to date, and to my daughter, Gavriela, who kept my spirits high. Countless conversations with my husband, Dan Burston, sparked many ideas that are reflected in these pages.

Sharna Olfman

I owe a debt of gratitude to many who played a role in assisting me in the scholarship leading up to this book's publication. Thank you to my coeditor and colleague at Point Park University, Sharna Olfman, for being the one who first alerted me to the growing problem of the over-medication of children. I am thankful as well to Dan Burston, who introduced me to the work of R. D. Laing and cultivated in me the critical thinking necessary to expose the hidden influences on psychiatry. Lisa Cosgrove and Robert Whitaker have been incredible sources of inspiration in their service as courageous role models for how to address pressing issues in a very public yet responsible way. I am grateful for the support and encouragement I have received from my colleagues at the Society for Humanistic Psychology (Division 32 of APA), including, among many others, Louis Hoffman, David Elkins, Shawn Rubin,

Richard Bargdill, Robert McInerney, Susan Gordon, Frank Farley, Kirk Schneider, Scott Churchill, Harris Friedman, and Fred Wertz. Thank you also to Mike Aquilina, Fr. Richard Infante, Don Fontana, and Sam Arnone for their spiritual guidance and encouragement. Of course, I would not have the time nor courage to take on all I do if it were not for the constant encouragement and support from my wife, April. Finally, my biggest debt of gratitude is owed to my mother, Diana Lewis, whose unconditional love and support has been the very literal foundation of all I have been able to accomplish in my life. Four years ago, in a series of events that will remain among the most tragic events in my life, she suffered a mental crisis and was heavily drugged on antipsychotics, suffered severe and debilitating side effects, and has yet to fully recover. I dedicate this book to her.

Brent Dean Robbins

Introduction

Sharna Olfman

The field of children's mental health has recently undergone a disturbing change. Market forces rather than medical research drive the practice of child psychiatry.[1] The profit motive has undermined even the most basic elements of safe and effective care. While giving children multiple psychiatric diagnoses and placing them on questionable polypharmacy regimens has been an accepted practice for some time,[2] the past decade has witnessed an alarming increase in the use of antipsychotics.

A landmark study conducted by Columbia University Professor Mark Olfson and his colleagues cataloged prescription rates of more than a million children covered by private insurance and revealed that since 2001 the number of antipsychotic prescriptions written for toddlers and preschoolers has doubled.[3] They also discovered that in a majority of cases, prescriptions were written to treat conditions for which the use of antipsychotic medication is neither FDA (Food and Drug Administration) approved nor justified by research, and mental health assessments were rarely conducted. While antipsychotic drug use among middle-class children has doubled, prescribing rates to low-income children covered by Medicaid have quadrupled.[4] Poor children are also more likely to receive an antipsychotic prescription from a pediatrician with no expertise in psychiatry and to have no recourse to psychotherapy. It is not only unethical but illegal for doctors billing under Medicaid to write off-label drug prescriptions for children and youth. This common practice has been largely ignored by the

mental health community, an issue that attorney and childhood advocate Jim Gottstein addresses in chapter 6.[5]

It is commonly believed that Medicaid favors drug therapies because
they are more cost effective and time effective than psychotherapies,
but neither claim is accurate. At $8 billion a year (and climbing), Med-
icaid now pays more for antipsychotic medication than for any other
category of drug, and once on an antipsychotic, withdrawal symptoms
make it not only difficult, but often dangerous to stop. Also, antipsychotics don't cure illness. They mask symptoms, and if the cause of the
symptoms isn't addressed, the child will not improve and drug use will
likely continue. Consequently, antipsychotics prescribed in childhood
often become a lifelong habit.[6] Clearly, these cradle-to-grave prescribing practices are a financial bonanza for the pharmaceutical industry.

DANGEROUS DRUGS

The antipsychotic drugs that are currently in use are referred to as
atypical to distinguish them from the original antipsychotic drugs developed in the 1950s for the treatment of adult schizophrenia. Atypical antipsychotics came on the market in the 1990s because the older
antipsychotics were no longer under patent and generic versions were
undercutting profits. The *new and improved* antipsychotics were introduced to the public through a well-orchestrated series of stories in the
media about the poor efficacy of the first generation of antipsychotic
medications, which were exposed as carrying a high risk of dangerous
side effects (although this was in fact known for decades). The atypical antipsychotics were widely touted as highly precise drugs for the
treatment of schizophrenia, with very few side effects.[7]

But these claims were not borne out in the research. A review of clinical trials involving more than 12,000 patients, which was published in
the *British Medical Journal* in 2000, found "no clear evidence that atypical
antipsychotics are more effective or better tolerated than conventional
antiypsychotics."[8] In fact, in the letter of approval to Janssen—the manufacturer of the atypical antipsychotic Risperdal—the FDA stated the
following:

We would consider any advertisement or promotional labeling for Risperdal false,
misleading, or lacking fair balance under 502 (a) and 502 (n) of the ACT if there is
presentation of data that conveys the impression that Risperdal [trade name for
risperidone] is superior to haloperidol or any other marketed antipsychotic drug
product with regard to safety or effectiveness.[9]

Furthermore, once Risperdal came on the market, researchers without ties to drug companies were free to test it, and study after study has

raised significant doubts about its safety and efficacy. Studies from Mc-Master University in Canada, the National Institute of Mental Health, and the University of Pittsburgh demonstrated that even a low dose of risperidone could cause Parkinsonism, akathisia, and extrapyramidal symptoms—the very same side effects associated with the first generation of antipsychotics. The prestigious medical journal the *Lancet* wrote a scathing review of the research practices that Janssen's researchers used to gain approval from the FDA and concluded that risperidone was a "marketing success, if nothing else."[10] But, lacking Janssen's PR budget, the *Lancet*'s findings were not aired in the media.

Similarly, though Eli Lilly's atypical antipsychotic drug olanzapine—which goes by the trade name Zyprexa—received FDA approval, 20 of the 2,500 patients who received olanzapine in clinical trials died. Twelve killed themselves, and two of the remaining eight deaths, from "aspiration pneumonia," were seen by FDA reviewers as possibly causally related to olanzapine. Twenty-two percent of the olanzapine patients suffered a serious adverse event. Two-thirds of the olanzapine patients didn't successfully complete the trials. More than one-fourth of the patients complained that the drug made them sleepy. Weight gain was a frequent problem, and other problems documented included Parkinson's akathisia, dystonia, hypotension, constipation, tachycardia, diabetic complications, seizures, increases in serum prolactin, liver abnormalities, and white blood cell disorders.[11] Paul Leber, the former director of the FDA's Division of Neuropharmacological Drugs, concluded that "no one should be surprised if, upon marketing, events of all kinds and severity not previously identified are reported in association with olanzapine's use."[12]

These very same atypical antipsychotics, initially marketed to adult schizophrenics, are now prescribed to millions of children across the United States. But, as award-winning journalist Robert Whitaker demonstrates in chapter 1, these drugs are even more injurious to children's developing brains and bodies.[13] Risperdal and its generic cousin risperidone account for three-quarters of the antipsychotics prescribed to children. Risperidone has proved to be such a dangerous drug that it is the subject of multiple lawsuits.[14] One side effect, which has prompted several of the lawsuits, is that it dramatically increases children's prolactin levels, resulting in numerous boys experiencing full breast development, necessitating mastectomies.[15]

OFF-LABEL PRESCRIPTIONS

Once a drug receives FDA approval, it can also be prescribed off label for *any* condition by *any* MD billing under private insurance, regardless of whether he or she is a mental health specialist. When a drug is used off label, its efficacy in treating the condition for which it was prescribed has not been proved. Atypical antipsychotics have been approved by the FDA for use with children to treat bipolar disorder, schizophrenia, and irritability associated with autism, but in a majority of cases, antipsychotics are prescribed to children to treat other conditions, such as attention-deficit/hyperactivity disorder (ADHD) and depression, or to control aggression and insomnia, though no sound research exists to support these applications.[16] Even where FDA approval for the use of antipsychotics with children has been granted, the research is scant, short-term, and, as we will see, of questionable validity.

MARKETING VERSUS EVIDENCE-BASED RESEARCH

The pharmaceutical industry has insinuated itself into every aspect of medical education, research, and practice. It provides the lion's share of funding for medical schools and hospitals, designs and implements drug research, supports medical journals through its advertising, and ghostwrites many lead articles. It heavily underwrites medical conferences and continuing education and bankrolls MDs, researchers, and even FDA employees. And it relentlessly markets its psychiatric drugs to mental health practitioners and the public at large. Even children are directly targeted by its marketing schemes through promotional materials such as coloring and picture books. As a consequence, psychiatric drug research and prevailing prescribing practices have become deeply enmeshed with the interests of pharmaceutical corporations, and they are thoroughly compromised as Gwen Olsen, a former pharmaceutical industry insider, reveals in chapter 4.[17]

The collusive relationship between psychiatry and the pharmaceutical industry compels us to scrutinize research that supports the use of psychotropic medication. We need to ask whether the researchers were in the employ of or received grants from any drug companies, whether the lead author actually conducted the research and wrote the article or whether his or her reputation was purchased, and what drug companies support the journals in which the research appears. A recent inquiry headed by Senator Charles Grassley, the ranking member of the Senate Finance Committee, revealed that Harvard professor Joseph Biederman—who almost single-handedly popularized the pediatric bipolar diagnosis received $1.6 million in undisclosed consulting fees from assorted drug companies. Even more damning, e-mail communications and slide presentations to Johnson & Johnson revealed that Biederman promised that his future research would "support the safety and effectiveness of their antipsychotic risperidone" in preschoolers.[18] It is impossible to overstate the cynicism entailed in creating a market among young children for a drug that is so perilous to their physical and neurological integrity.

GENERIC EFFECTS

In a perfect world, after the cause and course of an illness is understood, a medication is then designed to combat it with great specificity. This has virtually never been the case with psychiatric drugs, most of which were discovered by accident or through trial and error to mitigate some of the symptoms of a given psychiatric syndrome. Thorazine (chlorpromazine), the first drug to be marketed as an antipsychotic in the 1950s—was originally used as a surgical anesthetic. Its ability to calm the delusions and hallucinations of schizophrenic patients was stumbled upon by a surgeon who was using it to tranquilize a patient prior to surgery who just happened to be schizophrenic.[19] Antipsychotics were not *designed* to correct the alleged neurochemical imbalances that cause the psychotic and manic states associated with schizophrenia and bipolar disorder in the way that insulin treats diabetes. And marketing claims notwithstanding, the newer, atypical antipsychotics are no more precise than their older cousins that have fallen into such disrepute. Antipsychotics used to be referred to as major tranquilizers. They will, at least initially, calm an aggressive or agitated child. *Anyone* who takes an antipsychotic will be tranquilized.[20] But at the same time, they constitute such an assault to a child's body and brain that it is hard to fathom why they are being prescribed so widely and casually, when safer and more effective and humane treatment modalities already exist.

SIDELINING PROFESSIONAL PRACTICE

As antipsychotics become more widely prescribed by non-mental-health specialists, there has been a precipitous drop in thorough, thoughtful diagnostic assessments and access to psychotherapy.[21] It is unethical to prescribe an antipsychotic, or any psychiatric drug, without a comprehensive assessment. Prescribing a potent antipsychotic to a child without an assessment when other, more reliable methods of treatment are available is not only unethical, it is profoundly dehumanizing. When children act out or experience overwhelming fear, anger, or sadness, their behaviors and emotions are meaningful communications that need to be understood and addressed. Treating their actions and feelings as symptoms to be medicated away desensitizes us to the cause and depth of their suffering and denies them access to effective care.

In the 1980s, the children's mental health field witnessed the un-precedented rise in the use of stimulant medication. SSRI antidepres-sants became the drug of choice in the 1990s. Both classes of drugs are associated with a host of risk factors. In fact, SSRI antidepres-sant prescriptions to children now come with a black-box warning issued by the FDA that taking these drugs place children at a higher risk for suicide.[22] With each passing decade, the field of child psy-chiatry is careening wildly toward increasingly dangerous treatment regimens that now include drug cocktails and antipsychotics for pre-schoolers. Drugging our children offers a quick fix that relieves us of the challenging work of addressing complex and multifaceted cul-tural and environmental factors that are often the source of children's suffering.[23]

A CULTURE THAT HAS LOST ITS COMPASS

When children's cries for help are silenced by thoughtless and inap-propriate prescriptions that could tranquilize an elephant, we conve-niently ignore a host of social issues that undermine the integrity of families and children's mental health. The United States has the weak-est public policies among wealthy nations in support of family life. It is the only economically advantaged country that does not guaran-tee maternity leave to all women, and one of a handful of countries that does not subsidize and regulate its day cares. As a consequence, women who cannot afford to forgo a paycheck after giving birth are forced to rush back to work before they or their newborns are physi-cally or emotionally ready, while placing their infants in settings that offer substandard care. It does not take a degree in psychology to ap-preciate that this arrangement undermines the health of the mother who is still recovering from childbirth and robs parents and their chil-dren of a critically important opportunity to form secure and loving attachments. Other significant challenges to children's mental health include weak environmental protection policies that expose children to scores of neurotoxic chemicals, a public school system that privileges standardized testing over developmentally appropriate curricula, lim-ited opportunities for young children to play creatively in natural set-tings, and pervasive media that immerse children in sexualized and violent worlds while reducing their worth to a market share. Each of these issues, which I discuss at length in chapter 3, is complex and re-quires time and energy to address. But we can't eradicate their impact on children's health by giving them psychiatric drugs that numb their feelings and damage their brains.

FIXING THE PROBLEM

The psychiatric community is evidencing some awareness of its own culpability. The American Psychiatric Association recently revealed that it does not plan to include pediatric bipolar disorder (PBD) in its newest revision of the *Diagnostic and Statistical Manual* (*DSM*) due out in 2012,[24] a tacit acknowledgment that this diagnosis has been far too casually applied to children. The alleged symptom picture of PBD has no continuity with the symptoms of adult bipolar disorder, and research has shown that children assigned the PBD label are not developing into adults with bipolar disorder. However, plans are afoot to replace the PBD diagnosis with a new diagnostic category called temper disregulation disorder, an alleged brain disorder that has no research support and will likely generate as many drug sales as PBD. And so the impact of this change is cosmetic at best.

While it is necessary to hold child psychiatrists and pediatricians accountable for their prescribing practices, those of us who work in the mental health arena but do not have the mandate to prescribe drugs, including psychologists, social workers, and counselors, must examine our own responsibility to protect our young clients from harm. With increasing frequency, mental health professionals who may diagnose and treat but not medicate are referred children who have already begun a course of psychiatric medication or are scheduled to see a psychiatrist. If we feel that a child has been misdiagnosed and in consequence inappropriately prescribed an antipsychotic, or if we agree with the diagnosis but are aware of the harmful side effects of the medication, what legal and ethical considerations should guide our actions? These issues are addressed by psychologists Jacqueline Sparks and Barry Duncan in chapter 5 and attorney Jim Gottstein in chapter 6.

DRUGGING OUR CHILDREN

Drugging Our Children is divided into three parts. The first section articulates the problem in all of its complexity:

- the role of the pharmaceutical industry in creating a child market for antipsychotics
- the impact of antipsychotics on a child's developing brain and body
- the factors that have led the field of child psychiatry to make a devil's bargain with the pharmaceutical industry in its relentless promotion of antipsychotic medication as first-line treatment

- the ways in which American culture undermines children's healthy psychological development and foments the belief that the lion's share of children's behavioral and emotional issues are biochemical processes that can be fixed with a pill

The next section explores the legal and ethical ramifications of drugging our children. For example, what recourse do parents have if they believe that their child has been harmed by medication? What are the risks involved if they refuse to medicate their child? What ethical and legal rights and responsibilities do nonprescribing mental health practitioners have if they believe that a child in their care is being wrongfully medicated and harmed in the process?

The final section offers solutions that address the power of family and communities to foster and protect children's psychological development before problems arise or become entrenched, and it provides examples of effective interventions without recourse to antipsychotics. Child psychiatrist Tony Stanton shares more than a quarter of a century of experience in a residential setting, working with children who had cycled through multiple failed placements and were heavily medicated with drug cocktails that usually included antipsychotics when they first arrived. Social worker George Stone describes his decades of experience as a family therapist working with violent children, many of whom had been diagnosed as bipolar, who had already been prescribed, or were candidates for, antipsychotic medication. Psychologist Adena Meyers and her colleague Laura Berk, a leading expert in child development, remind us of the central role that parents can play in supporting their children's development and inoculating them against some of the psychological risk factors that we all inevitably face. And Stuart Shanker, an internationally known childhood expert, introduces a model of community intervention to proactively protect children's health and avoid the behavioral and emotional issues that lead to drugging.

When I began my research for this book, I believed that antipsychotics were dangerous drugs that were being recklessly prescribed to children but imagined that in rare instances, they were warranted. After immersing myself more deeply in the literature and the work of my fellow authors, I now share the viewpoint of my coeditor Brent Robbins that the risks that antipsychotics pose to children's minds and bodies far outweigh any conceivable benefits, and as such there should be a moratorium on antipsychotic prescriptions to all children. Many, but not all of the authors who have contributed to *Drugging Our Children* share this position. We are however, united in our belief that the cause and cure of children's psychological challenges are as complex and multifaceted as human nature itself, and tranquilizing children with antipsychotics who have no recourse to a thorough assessment and psychotherapy represents nothing less than malpractice. It is in my opinion a form of legally sanctioned child abuse. The authors who contributed to *Drugging Our Children* include some of America's leading childhood experts and advocates, and they are committed to putting an end to the rampant and irresponsible use of antipsycotic medication with children while promoting effective and humane mental health practice.

PART I

Drugging Our Children: The Problem

1

Weighing the Evidence: What Science Has to Say about Prescribing Atypical Antipsychotics to Children

Robert Whitaker

Today, prescribing antipsychotics to children and adolescents in the United States has become commonplace. More than 1 percent of American youth are on these medications for diagnoses that indicate long-term use. There is now enough scientific research describing how these drugs affect children and adolescents, both in terms of their safety and efficacy, and so we can now ask the key question: Are antipsychotics helping them to grow up and thrive as adults, or is it doing great harm?

THE RISE OF ANTIPSYCHOTIC PRESCRIPTIONS FOR CHILDREN

Prior to the early 1990s, it was uncommon to treat children with antipsychotics. Physicians understood that Thorazine, Haldol, and other neuroleptics were very problematic medications, and therefore prescribed them primarily to adults with schizophrenia or behavioral problems. For example, in 1987, among youth 6 to 17 years old covered by private insurance, only 1 in every 2,500 was prescribed an antipsychotic (0.04%). The prescribing rate for youth of that age covered by Medicaid was higher, and yet still uncommon (1 in 300).[1] There was virtually no prescribing of antipsychotics to children less than 6 years of age at that time. All told, there were fewer than 50,000 U.S. youth under 18 years old who were prescribed an antipsychotic in 1987.[2]

The first *atypical* antipsychotic to come to market in the United States was Clozaril in 1990. It was said to be an atypical antipsychotic because it didn't cause the motor dysfunction—known as extrapyramidal symptoms—that Thorazine and the other *standard* antipsychotics did. However, because Clozaril can cause agranulocytosis, a potentially fatal depletion of white blood cells, its use was reserved for refractory schizophrenia patients. Then Risperdal arrived on the market in 1993, an atypical touted as being much safer than the older antipsychotics and Clozaril. Other atypicals followed—Zyprexa, Seroquel, and so forth—said to be much safer as well.

It was this belief on the part of clinicians, that atypicals were safe, that made it possible for pharmaceutical companies to push their off-label use in pediatric populations. The drug companies worked closely with academic child psychiatrists in the United States to build this market. The manufacturers provided academic psychiatrists with research grants and paid them to serve as advisors, consultants, and speakers. Pharmaceutical companies refer to the academic doctors they hire as *thought leaders,* and in this instance, their thought leaders promoted the prescribing of atypicals for psychotic disorders, for juvenile bipolar disorder (which was rarely diagnosed prior to the arrival of the atypicals), and for controlling aggression and other behavioral problems.

The rise of juvenile bipolar illness is the best example of this market-building process. Up until the late 1970s, there was consensus among researchers that manic-depressive illness virtually never occurred in prepubertal children. But then physicians began to prescribe stimulants to children diagnosed with attention deficit disorder, a treatment that occasionally triggered manic (or psychotic) symptoms, and suddenly researchers began publishing case reports of younger children with manic-depressive illness (the researchers generally ignored the possibility that the stimulants had caused the mania). After Prozac and other SSRIs came to market in the late 1980s, the frequency of this diagnosis rose, as those drugs produce mania in children with some regularity. Together, prescriptions of stimulants and antidepressants to children and adolescents helped to create a new group of juvenile bipolar patients in the United States. However, when Risperdal came to market in 1993, there were still only 20,000 youth under age 20 so diagnosed.[3] Then, in 1996, Joseph Biederman, a child psychiatrist at Harvard-affiliated Massachusetts General Hospital, provided a new and greatly expanded diagnostic framework for juvenile bipolar disorder, and the juvenile bipolar boom was on.

In 2009, while giving a deposition in a legal case, Biederman acknowledged that there was no scientific discovery that led to his creation of this new diagnostic framework. Instead, he said, all psychiatric diagnoses "are subjective in children and in adults." As such, he and his colleagues had decided in 1996 that children with pronounced behavioral problems should be diagnosed with juvenile bipolar illness. "The conditions that we see in front of us are reconceptualized," he testified. "These children have been called in the past conduct disorder, oppositional-defiant disorder. It's not that these children did not exist, they were just under different names."[4] Biederman and his collaborators decided that "severe irritability" or "affective storms" would be the telltale sign of juvenile bipolar disorder. Having invented these new diagnostic criteria, they then announced that many children diagnosed with attention deficit/hyperactivity disorder (ADHD) were in fact "bipolar" or else "comorbid" for both illnesses.[5] The illness, Biederman told the public in the 1990s, was a "much more common condition than was previously thought," often appearing when children were only 4 or 5 years old.[6]

Biederman quickly became one of the pharmaceutical industry's favorite thought leaders. From 2000 to 2007, pharmaceutical companies paid him $1.6 million for his various services.[7] In addition, Janssen pharmaceutical company, the division of Johnson & Johnson that sells Risperdal, gave Biederman $2 million to create the Johnson & Johnson Center for Pediatric Psychopathology at Massachusetts General Hospital.[8] The center, Biederman wrote in a 2002 report, was a "strategic collaboration" that would "move forward the commercial goals of J&J." He and his colleagues promised to develop "screening tests" for juvenile bipolar illness, and to conduct continuing medical education courses to train pediatricians and psychiatrists to use their new diagnostic tool. Their work, Biederman wrote, would "alert physicians to the existence of a large group of children who might benefit from treatment with Risperdal." In addition, the center would promote the understanding that "pediatric mania evolves into what some have called mixed or atypical mania in adulthood, [which] will provide further support for the chronic use of Risperdal from childhood through adulthood."[9]

Thanks in large part to Biederman's efforts, the number of U.S. children under age 20 diagnosed with bipolar disorder soared from 20,000 in 1994 to 800,000 in 2003, a 40-fold increase.[10] It has continued to rise since then. The number of atypical antipsychotic prescriptions to children under age 18 in the United States doubled from about 2.2 million in 2003 to 4.4 million in 2006. "The expanded use of bipolar disorder as a pediatric diagnosis has made children the fastest-growing part of the $11.5 billion U.S. market for antipsychotic drugs," Bloomberg News reported in 2007.[11]

As a result of this extraordinary explosion of pediatric bipolar diagnoses, today antipsychotics are prescribed to more than 1 percent of all

U.S. youth under 18 years old, and only a small percentage of this use is to treat schizophrenia and other psychotic disorders. In a 2006 study, researchers found that 38 percent of antipsychotic prescriptions to children were for disruptive behaviors, 32 percent for mood disorders, 17 percent for developmental disorders or mental retardation, and 14 percent for psychotic disorders.[12] The drugs are now being used for an ever broadening range of conditions, including ADHD, impulsivity, insomnia, posttraumatic stress disorder, obsessive-compulsive symptoms, eating disorders, and—as one researcher put it—poor tolerance of "frustration."[13]

HOW ATYPICAL ANTIPSYCHOTICS ACT ON THE BRAIN

During the past 20 years, the public has regularly been told that psychiatric medications fix "chemical imbalances" in the brain, and therefore are like "insulin for diabetes." When the atypical antipsychotics came to market, the National Alliance on Mental Illness, in a book titled *Breakthroughs in Antipsychotic Medications,* informed readers that these new drugs "do a better job (than the old ones) of balancing all of the brain chemicals, including dopamine and serotonin."[14] As a result, much of the public has come to believe that when atypicals are prescribed for juvenile bipolar illness and for other childhood disorders, the drugs are somehow correcting something known to be amiss in the brain. But, as a review of the science shows, that isn't true.

In the 1970s, researchers discovered that Thorazine and other antipsychotics blocked dopamine receptors in the brain, and in particular a subtype known as D2 receptors. At a therapeutic dose, these drugs block 70 percent of the D2 receptors. With this understanding, researchers then hypothesized that schizophrenia was caused by too much dopamine activity in the brain. But when they investigated that hypothesis in the 1970s and 1980s, they did not find that schizophrenia patients had, as a matter of course, *hyperactive* dopamine systems. As Harvard University neuroscientist Steven Hyman explained in a 2002 textbook, *Molecular Neuropharmacology,* "there is no compelling evidence that a lesion in the dopamine system is a primary cause of schizophrenia."[15]

However, these investigations did not consider how the brain reacts to an antipsychotic. Nerve cells or neurons communicate in this way: A presynaptic neuron releases a chemical messenger (such as dopamine) into the tiny gap between neurons known as the synaptic cleft, and this molecule then binds with receptors on the surface of the postsynaptic neuron. The neurotransmitter is said to fit into the receptor like a key into a lock. Thorazine and other standard antipsychotics gum up the D2 locks, so to speak, and in this manner inhibit the firing of the postsynaptic neurons. This blockade thwarts the transmission of messages along dopaminergic pathways in the brain, which are essential to the functioning of the basal ganglia, the limbic system, and the frontal lobes. In response, the brain goes through a series of compensatory adaptations. For a time, the presynaptic neurons release more dopamine than normal, while the postsynaptic neurons increase the density of their D2 receptors by 30 percent or more. These adaptations are designed to keep the dopaminergic pathways at least somewhat functional. The first compensatory adaptation appears to break down after a while, but the increase in D2 receptors remains and can be detected at autopsy.

While risperidone (Risperdal), olanzapine (Zyprexa), quetiapine (Seroquel), and other newer antipsychotics are grouped together as atypicals, they vary considerably in their pharmacological effects, and thus are more accurately described as *second generation antipsychotics* (SGAs). They are all broad-acting agents. While they may not block D2 receptors quite as potently as Thorazine and the other first-generation antipsychotics (FGAs), they may also bind with serotonergic, histaminergic, adrenergic, and muscarinic receptors.[16] For the most part, atypicals thwart the passage of messages along these various neuronal pathways, triggering an avalanche of compensatory adaptations in the brain.

The drugs' disruption of normal functioning along these various neuronal pathways causes many predictable adverse events. Since dopaminergic pathways are involved in the control of motor movements, drugs that block dopamine receptors can cause Parkinsonian symptoms, muscle dystonias, akathisia, prolactin increase, and sexual dysfunction. Blocking serotonergic receptors can cause an increase in appetite, weight gain, and metabolic changes associated with an increased risk of diabetes. Blocking muscarinic M1 receptors can cause memory and cognition problems. And so on . . . each neurotransmitter has its own side effect profile.[17]

Moreover, these are the *predictable* side effects. Any drug that blocks multiple types of receptors can be expected to cause many unexpected adverse events too.

There are also distinct withdrawal effects associated with the different neuronal pathways. For instance, if a drug blocks D2 receptors, the withdrawal of that drug may lead to psychosis, mania, agitation, and akathisia. If a drug blocks muscarinic M1 receptors, its withdrawal may cause agitation, confusion, anxiety, and insomnia. And so on . . . withdrawal effects from a psychiatric drug may vary according to which neuronal pathways have been altered by it.[18] (See Table 1.1.)

TABLE 1.1. Expected Effects from a Drug's Blockade of Receptors

Receptor Type	Adverse Events	Withdrawal Effects
Dopamine	EPS, weight gain, endocrine effects, akathisia, tardive dyskinesia, increased prolactin, sexual or reproductive system dysfunction	Psychosis, mania, agitation, akathisia, dyskinesia
Serotonin	Weight gain, diabetes, increased appetite	EPS, akathisia, psychosis, decreased appetite
Histamine	Weight gain, diabetes, sedation	Agitation, insomnia, anxiety, EPS
Muscarinic	Dry mouth, blurred vision, constipation, urinary retention, diabetes, memory problems cognitive problems, tachycardia, hypertension	Agitation, confusion, psychosis, anxiety, insomnia, sialorrhea, EPS, akathisia, diarrhea, nausea, vomiting, bradycardia, hypotension, syncope
Adrenergic	Postural hypotension, dizziness, syncope	Tachycardia, hypertension, hypotension, dizziness

EPS = extrapyramidal symptoms.
Source: C Correll, "Assessing and maximizing the safety and tolerability of antipsychotics used in the treatment of children and adolescents." *J Clin Psychiatry* 69, suppl. 4 (2008): 26–36. Also see C. Correll, "Antipsychotic use in children and adolescents." *J Am Acad Child Adolesc Psychiatry* 47 (2008):9–20.

Thus, once a child or youth begins taking an antipsychotic, the child can be expected to experience many adverse events while on the drug, and to experience many distressing symptoms when trying to go off it.

THE EFFICACY OF SECOND GENERATION ANTIPSYCHOTICS IN CHILDREN AND ADOLESCENTS

The hope with any drug is that its benefit will outweigh the risks associated with its use. Because Risperdal and the other SGAs are so broad acting, they are bound to cause many adverse effects. As such, they should produce a marked therapeutic benefit of some type in children so that their use—when the risks and benefits are tallied up—can be assessed as helpful.

Short-Term Use

The FDA approved Risperdal and the other SGAs based on the results from industry-funded, short-term studies with adult schizophrenia patients. The pharmaceutical companies then promoted their off-label use in pediatric populations. Eventually, the pharmaceutical companies funded trials of their SGAs in children and adolescents, and the results from those studies led the FDA to approve Risperdal, Zyprexa, Seroquel, and Abilify for schizophrenia, bipolar disorder, and irritability in autism.[19]

In a 2010 review of the published literature, Spanish investigators found reports of nine "placebo-controlled, randomized studies" of those four SGAs in children with psychotic and bipolar spectrum disorders. The industry-funded trials lasted from three to eight weeks. While the placebo patients in the trials saw their symptoms improve, the patients treated with one of the atypicals improved to a greater extent. As such, those industry-funded trials were seen as proving the efficacy of the four drugs for youth under 18 years old.[20]

However, when the National Institute of Mental Health (NIMH) conducted its TEOSS study of antipsychotics for early onset schizophrenia in youth 8 to 19 years old, the efficacy of the two SGAs that were tested was much more muted. The 116 youth enrolled in the trial were randomized to molindone (an FGA), Risperdal, or Zyprexa, and at the end of eight weeks, the response rate was 50 percent for those treated with molindone, 46 percent for those treated with Risperdal, and 34 percent for Zyprexa. Only 31 of the 76 youth treated with a SGA "responded" to the drug.[21]

Unfortunately, the TEOSS trial was not placebo controlled, and so it is impossible to know how those response rates would compare to outcomes in nonmedicated youth. Furthermore, in this trial, many of the patients were on other psychiatric medications (in addition to the antipsychotic), which obviously confounded the efficacy results. Those who were on antidepressants and mood stabilizers prior to the study were allowed to continue on those drugs, and during the eight-week trial, many of the children were prescribed drugs—anticholinergic agents, propranolol, and benzodiazepines—to counter the side effects of the antipsychotic agents. Given the lack of a placebo control and the use of these other psychotropic agents, this one government-funded trial of the SGAs provides no evidence that they are an effective short-term treatment for early onset schizophrenia.

Additional evidence for the short-term use of SGAs in pediatric populations consists of a handful of randomized studies that showed several of the drugs to be effective for controlling aggression and other disruptive behaviors (studies often conducted in children with autism).[22] Since antipsychotics are often sedating and may curb both motor movement and emotional engagement, the finding that SGAs are effective in curbing aggressive behavior over the short term was to be expected. The FGAs have long been used in zoos for such purposes.

Although the FDA has approved four SGAs for pediatric use, European and Canadian regulatory authorities have been much more cautious about giving their regulatory blessing for use of these agents in children. As of 2010, the only SGA licensed in Europe as an *antipsychotic* for pediatric use was Abilify (for schizophrenia patients 15 to 17 years old).[23] In several European countries, Risperdal is licensed for treating children with severe disruptive disorders (but not as an antipsychotic).[24] As of 2009, Health Canada had not approved any SGA for pediatric use.[25]

Long-Term Use

In the TEOSS study, those who initially responded to the drug (54 of 116 patients) were then followed for an additional 44 weeks. As the TEOSS investigators noted, theirs was the first well-designed study that sought to assess the effectiveness and safety of SGAs in juveniles for as long as one year. Unfortunately, the antipsychotics failed this test. In the 44-week drug-maintenance study, 40 of the 54 youth dropped out, mostly because of "adverse effects" or "inadequate response." Moreover, during this 44-week follow-up, those treated with Risperdal worsened *significantly* in their functional capacities, while those treated with Zyprexa worsened slightly in this regard. (There was no change in functioning in the molindone group.) In addition, the psychotic symptoms of the children treated with Risperdal or Zyprexa worsened to a small extent during the follow-up.[26]

Here, then, are the bottom-line results from the TEOSS study. Only 14 of the original cohort of 116 patients (12%) responded to an antipsychotic and then stayed on the drug and in the trial throughout the 44-week maintenance study. The remaining 102 children (88%) either failed to respond to an antipsychotic or dropped out during the maintenance period, mostly because of adverse effects or because they worsened on the drug. The NIMH researchers drew the obvious bottom-line conclusion: "Few youths with early onset schizophrenia who are treated with antipsychotic medications for up to a year appear to benefit from their initial treatment choice over the long-term."[27]

Unfortunately, since this longer-term trial wasn't placebo controlled, it doesn't provide any insight into how unmedicated patients might have fared at the end of one year. But in the industry-funded trials, the children treated with placebo did improve over the short term, and it is reasonable to think that such children might continue to improve if given some type of nondrug care for a longer period of time. Yet—and this shows the utter deficiency of the evidence base for prescribing SGAs to children—there has not been any study that has looked at that possibility.

As this review of the literature shows, there is no evidence that SGAs provide a benefit—in terms of symptom reduction and improvement in functioning compared to placebo—for *any* disorder at the end of one year. As such, in the risk-benefit analysis for long-term use, there is no positive finding that can be chalked up on the benefit side of the ledger. What remains then is to look at the harm these agents can cause.

EVIDENCE OF HARM DONE

Because the SGAs may act on a number of different neurotransmitter pathways, and may do so with varying degrees of potency, the adverse effects that the individual drugs cause can vary widely. But as a class of drugs, the SGAs cause a dizzying array of physical, emotional, and cognitive problems.

Movement Disorders

Although the SGAs may be less likely than the older antipsychotics to cause motor problems (extrapyramidal symptoms, or EPS), they still cause these problems with considerable frequency. In the one double-blind, randomized study that directly compared EPS rates with an FGA and SGAs in youth under 18 years old, 67 percent of the haloperidol group experienced "substantial EPS," versus 56 percent of those given Zyprexa and 53 percent of the Risperdal group.[28] While there have been a number of published studies reporting very low EPS rates in children treated with SGAs, those findings often have come from industry-funded studies of children with autism, with the autistic children having to "spontaneously report" that they were experiencing motor problems.[29]

The SGAs may also cause akathisia, a painful inner agitation associated with an increased risk of suicide and homicide. Five percent to 20 percent of pediatric patients may experience this side effect in a short trial.[30]

The published rates of tardive dyskinesia (TD) in children and adolescents treated with SGAs vary widely. TD is characterized by rhythmic involuntary motor movements, such as a constant licking of the lips, and often the abnormal movements don't go away even if the antipsychotic is withdrawn, which is evidence that the basal ganglia has been permanently damaged. In short industry-funded studies, researchers have reported seeing almost no cases of TD in their pediatric patients. However, TD is a condition that usually develops with longer exposure to antipsychotics, and two studies that looked at longer-term SGA use in children reported TD rates similar to what is seen in adult patients taking FGAs. Researchers at the University of Maryland

School of Medicine reported that 3 percent of the 116 pediatric patients they studied developed TD within 6 to 12 months on an SGA, and that 10 percent did so after being on the drugs for one to two years.[31] Spanish investigators reported an even higher rate: They determined that 38 percent of children and adolescents on antipsychotics for longer than one year showed signs of mild TD.[32] Fortunately, it appears that TD is more likely to disappear in pediatric patients than in adult patients if the offending antipsychotic is withdrawn, and thus, in this age group, the initial appearance of TD symptoms may not mean that the damage to the basal ganglia is beyond repair.

Metabolic Dysfunction

All SGAs can cause weight gain, with Zyprexa the worst offender in this regard. In a 6-month study of first-episode psychotic patients, the Zyprexa-treated youth gained an average of 34 pounds.[33] Israeli physicians reported that 90 percent of youth taking Zyprexa and 43 percent of those on Risperdal gained more than 7 percent of their baseline weight within 12 weeks.[34] When investigators at Cincinnati Children's Hospital and British Columbia Children's Hospital in Vancouver surveyed their juvenile patients with exposure to SGAs, they found that more than 50 percent were overweight or obese.[35] This weight gain, which is obviously problematic from a physical standpoint, may also cause pediatric patients to become depressed and suffer from low-esteem.[36]

The SGAs can also cause diabetes, which is one of the reasons that Eli Lilly and other SGA makers have been successfully sued for their off-label marketing of these agents to children. In 2010, Canadian investigators reported that 22 percent of pediatric patients treated with SGAs at a children's hospital in British Columbia had "impaired fasting glucose and or type 2 diabetes."[37] Since fat tissue can increase insulin resistance and glucose intolerance, this diabetes risk may be secondary to the weight gain. However, it appears that SGAs may also directly impair pancreatic beta-cell function and promote insulin resistance in that way.[38]

SGAs commonly cause a significant increase in triglycerides and LDL-cholesterol (dyslipidemia). In a survey of 95 juvenile inpatients at Cincinnati Children's Hospital who had been treated with an SGA for longer than 1 month, 51 percent had developed dyslipidemia.[39]

The weight gain, glucose intolerance, and dyslipidemia are all evidence that an SGA may profoundly impair the body's metabolic system. If a pediatric patient becomes obese and develops two other signs of metabolic dysfunction (high blood pressure, dyslipidemia, or high fasting glucose), the patient is said to have developed a "metabolic syndrome." In their 2010 study, Canadian investigators determined that 27 percent of juvenile patients treated with an SGA on average for 12 months suffered from this broader level of metabolic dysfunction.[40]

The weight gain and metabolic impairment puts the pediatric patient on a path toward poor long-term physical health and ultimately early death. "Because drug-induced metabolic changes can persist over time and may not be fully reversible upon drug discontinuation, the implications for distal health outcomes can be profound," wrote the NIMH's Benedetto Vitiello in 2009. "Age-inappropriate weight gain and obesity increase the risk for a variety of negative outcomes, such as diabetes, hyperlipidemia, and hypertension, which are major risk factors for cardiovascular diseases and reduced quality of life and life expectancy."[41]

Endocrine Dysfunction

Several news stories reported on teenage boys prescribed Risperdal who have grown breasts and even begun lactating. This is because Risperdal may dramatically increase prolactin levels (and thus cause hyperolactinemia). While Risperdal is more likely than the other SGAs to cause this hormonal disruption, Spanish investigators reported in 2007 that 49 percent of youth treated with an SGA for longer than a year had hyperolactinemia.[42] This can cause breast enlargement and hypogonadism in males, and galactorrhea, amenorrhea, and hirsutism in females. Elevated prolactin levels may also cause a decrease in libido, sexual dysfunction, and decreased bone density. The bone density deficiency "may not be recovered later in life," and thus the SGA-treated child may end up with a lifelong increased risk of bone fractures.[43]

Other Adverse Effects

Researchers have reported that SGAs can occasionally cause elevated levels of liver enzymes in pediatric patients.[44] The cardiovascular risks associated with SGAs include cardiomegaly, tachycardia, arrhythmia, QTc prolongation, heart disease not otherwise specified, and high blood pressure.[45] In industry-funded trials, the reported adverse events included dizziness, facial flushing, dry mucous membranes, decreased sweating, constipation, urinary retention, headaches, blurred vision, and tinnitus.[46] Cases of neuroleptic malignant syndrome and pancreatitis, both of which can be fatal, have been reported in pediatric patients.[47]

SGAs can also cause an array of emotional and cognitive problems. In the TEOSS study, 26 percent of the patients reported being anxious.[48]

Other common side effects include irritability, depression, emotional lethargy, and decreased concentration.[49] SGAs are also sedating drugs, with more than half of the pediatric patients in some trials complaining of this effect, which is associated with "cognitive impairment and decreased mental activity."[50]

Poor Global Health

As can be seen from this review of adverse effects, the SGAs profoundly impair a child's physical, cognitive, and emotional well-being. While the percentage of children and adolescents who suffer any particular adverse effect may vary, nearly all children treated with an SGA will suffer an adverse effect of some type. The TEOSS investigators reported that 83 percent of the patients in the follow-up study suffered an "adverse" event.[51] Similarly, in a survey of 4,140 Medicaid youth treated with SGAs for longer periods of time, University of South Carolina researchers found that 47 percent suffered from digestive or urogenital problems; 36 percent had skin, musculoskeletal, or respiratory conditions; 9 percent had cardiovascular disorders; and 3 percent had diabetes. "The treated cohort exhibits a high incidence and diverse array of treatment-related adverse events," they concluded.[52]

LONG-TERM BRAIN DAMAGE

Although it may be that tardive dyskinesia is largely reversible when it first develops in children and adolescents, that return to health is likely to happen only if the offending SGA is withdrawn. But once youth are on SGAs, withdrawing from the drugs can be difficult, and often when youth experience problems on an SGA, they are then prescribed other psychiatric medications to go along with the antipsychotic, and thus they end up on drug cocktails. Given this common practice, it is reasonable to think that when researchers—at some point in the future—assess how children are doing after five years or more on an SGA, they will find high rates of TD, and that it will be much less reversible than it is in youth who have been on an SGA for only a few months.

In adults, the fact that TD often doesn't go away after the offending neuroleptic is withdrawn is evidence that the basal ganglia, which is the area of the brain that controls motor movement, has been permanently damaged. Adults who develop TD also show signs of a global decline in brain function. Researchers have determined that TD is associated with emotional disengagement, psychosocial impairment, and a decline in memory, visual retention, and the capacity to learn.[53] People with severe TD, one investigator concluded, lose their "road map to consciousness."[54]

In addition, there is now good evidence that both FGAs and SGAs shrink the brain, and that this shrinkage is associated with functional impairment and cognitive decline. In 1989, Nancy Andreasen, who was editor-in-chief of the *American Journal of Psychiatry* from 1993 to 2005, began a long-term study of more than 500 schizophrenia patients. She periodically measured their brain volumes with magnetic resonance scans, and in articles published in 2003 and 2005, she reported "progressive brain volume reductions" in her patients. This brain shrinkage, she found, was associated with increased emotional disengagement, functional impairment, and cognitive decline.[55]

In those 2003 and 2005 reports, Andreasen attributed the brain shrinkage to the disease, a pathological process that antipsychotics couldn't arrest. "The medications currently used cannot modify an injurious process occurring in the brain, which is the underlying basis of symptoms," she wrote in her 2003 paper. However, even as she was publishing those findings, other research—in animals and schizophrenia patients—indicated that the drugs might exacerbate this brain shrinkage (or be the primary cause of it). For instance, in a 2005 study of macaque monkeys, a daily dose of haloperidol or Zyprexa for 18 months led to an 8 percent to 11 percent reduction "in mean fresh brain weight" compared to controls.[56]

In 2011, Andreasen reported that the brain shrinkage in her schizophrenia patients was indeed drug related. She found that long-term use of FGAs, SGAs, and Clozaril was "associated with smaller brain tissue volumes," and that this shrinkage is dose related. The more of a drug a person is given, she wrote, the greater the "association with smaller grey matter volumes." Similarly, the "progressive decrement in white matter volume was most evident among patients who received more antipsychotic treatment." Finally, she determined that this shrinkage "occurs independent of illness severity and substance abuse." Those two factors—illness severity and substance abuse—had "minimal or no effects" on brain volumes.[57]

Andreasen's published articles convincingly tell of an iatrogenic process. Long-term use of an antipsychotic causes the brain to shrink, and as this occurs, the person's ability to think and function in the world declines. When children are placed on SGAs, this brain shrinkage will begin at an early age.

EARLY DEATH

Since the introduction of the SGAs, the mortality rate for schizophrenia patients has notably worsened.[58] In addition, a 2006 study found that the seriously mentally ill are now dying 15 to 25 years earlier than normal.[59] They are dying from cardiovascular ailments, respiratory problems, metabolic illness, diabetes, kidney failure, and so forth—the physical ailments pile up as people stay on antipsychotics for years on end.

This early death is showing up in adults who were first treated with psychiatric medications when they were in their 20s or 30s. However, the children and adolescents being put on SGAs today will have years of exposure to these drugs by the time they reach their early 20s, which raises an obvious question: How much longer will they live on these agents? Will many die in their 30s? Early 40s? Fifteen to 20 years from now, reports in the scientific literature will provide us with the answer, and given what is known about these drugs, we can expect that the news will be grim.

WEIGHING ALL THE EVIDENCE

Such is the story that science tells about prescribing atypical antipsychotics to children and adolescents. In industry-funded trials, four SGAs were found to be effective over the short term in curbing the symptoms of schizophrenia and mania, and for curbing aggression and other disruptive behaviors in certain pediatric populations. However, in the one study funded by the NIMH, fewer than half of the patients responded to an antipsychotic in the short term, and at the end of 12 months, only 12 percent of the children were still on the initial antipsychotic, either because of side effects or because the drug didn't work.

The SGAs work by interfering with the normal functioning of multiple neurotransmitters, which is why they cause so many adverse effects. These drugs may impair metabolic, hormonal, muscular, and cardiovascular functions. Yet, once on an atypical, a younger person may have difficulty getting off the drug because of withdrawal effects, and so initial use often leads to long-term use, with the young patient ending up on a drug cocktail.

Those that stay on SGAs long term, into adulthood, can expect their lives to be diminished in multiple ways. They likely will suffer from poor physical health, and over time, as their brains shrink, their ability to function in society—their capacity to emotionally engage with others and to think—will diminish. They can expect to die quite early.

We can now return to the question raised at the beginning of this chapter. Does prescribing atypicals to children and adolescents help them to grow up and thrive as adults? Or is it doing great harm? Science provides a clear—and tragic—answer to that question.

2

From Ice Pick Lobotomies to Antipsychotics as Sleep Aids for Children: A Historical Perspective

Brent Dean Robbins

Twenty-five percent of American children and 30 percent of adolescents take drugs for chronic medical illness, and a majority of these prescriptions are for psychiatric conditions.[1] Antipsychotic medication is the fastest-growing category. Since 2001, the prescription rate of atypical antipsychotics for pediatric populations has doubled. As one commentator put it, "We either have the sickest pediatric population in the world, or there is something very wrong with the way therapies are driven in our health care system."[2]

The 40-fold increase in the diagnosis of pediatric bipolar disorder (PBD) that we witnessed this past decade is what initially drove prescriptions of antipsychotics to children.[3] Over the past few years, however, antipsychotics are being prescribed to children for a growing number of psychiatric diagnoses and symptoms including pervasive developmental disorder, mental retardation, attention-deficit/hyperactivity disorder (ADHD), and disruptive behavior disorder.[4] Children between the ages of 2 and 5 are the fastest-growing market for antipsychotics.[5] Among hospitalized children and adolescents, as many as 44 percent of pediatric patients are prescribed antipsychotic medications.[6]

The striking increase in antipsychotic prescriptions for children and adolescents is cause for grave concern because of the severe and potentially irreversible side effects associated with this class of drugs, as Robert Whitaker describes in chapter 1. The combined risks of rapid weight gain and metabolic disturbance posed by antipsychotics place children at risk for type 2 diabetes[7]—a fact that may help explain the lockstep increase in type 2 diabetes and antipsychotic use. Irreversible motor disorders, including tardive dyskinesia (involuntary tics) and akathisia (constant agitation and inability to sit still) are commonly found with long-term use.[8] Antipsychotic medications also shorten life expectancy and cause deterioration of the brain—the extent of which is correlated with the strength of the prescription.[9]

In spite of these disturbing side effects, an argument could still be made for prescribing antipsychotics to children if they were effective in curing disease, and if their use was limited to the most debilitating diagnoses and symptoms. But neither is the case. As Whitaker has documented in *Anatomy of an Epidemic,* antipsychotic use is more likely to *cause* rather than cure long-term mental disability.[10] And increasingly, antipsychotics are being prescribed for casual symptoms rather than serious illness. Seroquel, for example, is commonly prescribed to children as a sleep aid![11]

As dangerous as they are on their own, antipsychotics are frequently prescribed to children as part of a drug cocktail. The risks entailed in prescribing multiple psychiatric drugs to children are poignantly illustrated by the tragic story of Rebecca Riley.[12] Rebecca was only 28 months old when a highly respected psychiatrist diagnosed her with PBD and ADHD. Rebecca was prescribed a combination of Depakote, an antiseizure drug; Clonidine, an antihypertensive; and Seroquel, an antipsychotic. On December 13, 2006, 4-year-old Rebecca Riley died of a prescription drug overdose.

Contrast Rebecca's case to Kyle Warren's whose story was highlighted in a 2010 issue of the *New York Times.*[13] Like Riley, Kyle was also treated for behavioral problems, which manifested as intense temper tantrums that his mother found difficult to manage. Between 18 months and 3 years of age, Kyle's pediatrician prescribed him Risperdal, an antipsychotic; Prozac, an antidepressant; a stimulant; and several sleep medications. He did not refer the family for psychotherapy to help resolve his temper tantrums but instead moved directly to powerful drugs. Kyle could do little more than sleep, drool, and overeat, and he quickly ballooned up to a dangerous weight. His mother, Brandy Warren, had enough sense to seek a second opinion, and fortunately entered Kyle into a program at Tulane University, which gradually weaned him off the meds. Once he was relatively medication free, with the exception of a stimulant for ADHD, he began to show rapid improvement in his performance in school, and his charming personality began to emerge, to the delight of his mother.

Rebecca Riley's death is a cautionary tale that underscores the extent to which toddlers and children are being recklessly diagnosed with serious mental illness and prescribed combinations of dangerous drugs.

Ellen Leibenluf at the National Institute of Mental Health (NIMH) has persuasively demonstrated that most kids who are diagnosed as bipolar in childhood do not in fact have bipolar disorder. Children diagnosed with bipolar disorder who she followed into adulthood did not as a rule become bipolar adults. In a majority of cases, their diagnosis was changed to anxiety or depression.[14] Why are so many children being wrongfully diagnosed and unnecessarily medicated at younger and younger ages? One part of the problem is that, in many cases, pediatricians are failing to do an adequate job. Recent research has shown that, in a majority of cases, children prescribed antipsychotics were never properly assessed, never referred for psychotherapy, and never saw a psychiatrist.[15] Although 72 percent of pediatricians prescribe psychotropics, only 8 percent report having adequate training in prescribing them, and only 16 percent felt comfortable about prescribing them to their patients.[16] These statistics are all the more worrisome in light of predictions that in the near future, the treatment of mental illness could take up as much as 40 percent of a pediatrician's practice.[17] Another closely related problem is that for every 1,000–2,000 children diagnosed with a mental illness in the United States, it is estimated that that there is only one pediatric psychiatrist[18]—a ratio that is very troubling, to say the least. However, the dearth of pediatric psychiatrists does not tell the full story of the rise in psychiatric diagnoses and antipsychotic drug prescriptions among children.

Poor and disadvantaged children are the ones most at risk for inept clinical care and overmedication. According to research funded by the federal government, children covered by Medicaid are four times more likely to be prescribed antipsychotic medication compared to their privately insured peers.[19] Children in custody of the state who are in state-run jails or residential programs are especially at risk of being heavily medicated on antipsychotics. In 2011, the Head of Florida's Department of Juvenile Justice initiated an investigation into the overuse of antipsychotics among juveniles in state custody.[20] The evidence clearly showed that antipsychotics were among the most commonly prescribed medications, often for reasons that were not approved by the FDA. To get a sense of the magnitude of antipsychotic prescriptions ordered by the state, records from 2007 revealed that the Department of Juvenile Justice purchased double the amount of Seroquel as compared to Ibuprofen! In a two-year span, the Department of Juvenile Justice purchased 326,081 tablets of antipsychotics including Seroquel, Abilify, and Risperdal.[21]

Youth in foster care are also at high risk of being prescribed antipsychotic medication. Children in foster care who are covered by Medicaid are three times more likely to be prescribed psychiatric medications compared to their peers from low-income families on Medicaid who are not in foster care.[22] Boys under the age of 12 and nonwhite children are especially at risk for being medicated.[23] Even among the privately insured, children between the ages of 2 and 5 are being heavily targeted for antipsychotic use.[24]

The sharp rise in psychiatric diagnoses and psychiatric drug use among our youth is a clarion call to address something fundamentally wrong with our culture. What exactly has gone wrong? In the next chapter, Sharna Olfman examines the ways in which contemporary society is failing to address children's essential needs. Here, I focus on several key moments in the history of psychiatry that reveal otherwise opaque socioeconomic forces that influence current practice. Bringing these issues to light can lead to more creative solutions with which to solve the epidemic of children's psychiatric diagnoses and the rampant use of dangerous drugs.

LESSONS FROM HISTORY, PART 1: PSYCHIATRY AND EUGENICS

Most histories of psychiatry begin with a lurid description of England's infamous Bethlehem Hospital. From the 12th through the 17th centuries, across Europe, the mentally ill were generally viewed as wild animals that needed to be broken in order to be tamed. This frame of mind helps to explain the brutality with which the mentally ill were treated by their alleged caretakers. It was common for physicians to not only restrain patients with chains, but to submit them to a host of ordeals including bleeding, emetics, and blistering.

Benjamin Rush is considered to be the Father of American Psychiatry. In the early 1800s, he was one of the first mental health specialists to conceptualize mental illness as a biological illness as opposed to "possession of demons," and he was appalled by the inhumane treatment of the mentally ill to that point. However, his misguided belief that mental illness was caused by disruptions of blood circulation led to tortuous "cures" such as being strapped to a "tranquilizer chair"—a fate that at least one patient had to endure for six months.[25]

Despite the brutish origins of modern psychiatry, the harsh treatment of patients began to subside by the late 18th century to be replaced by a more humane approach, *moral therapy*. The York Retreat in England, established in 1796 by William Tuke, was a Quaker-operated religious hospice that is considered to be the birthplace of *moral treatment*.[26] The approach was soon adopted in the United States in places such as Hartford Retreat, McLean Hospital, and Bloomingdale Asylum. This approach to treatment has been credited as the first attempt to conceptualize and treat mental illness using psychological concepts and interventions. While the treatment was anchored to religious presuppositions, it also relied on evidence of the efficacy of treatment, which marks the beginning of a scientific approach. In contrast to the inhumane treatment that the mentally ill had previously been subjected to, consistent with the nonviolent philosophy of the Quakers, William Tuke focused on the healing powers of benevolence and charity. Patients were understood to have an innate capacity to heal, and the environment was structured to reduce stress and strain in order to promote the patient's recovery.

Moral treatment was remarkably successful in its time. In *Mad in America*, Whitaker reports on some of the impressive findings during treatments in this era:

Hartford Retreat announced that twenty-one of twenty-three patients admitted in its first three years recovered with this gentle treatment. At McLean Hospital, 59 percent of the 732 patients admitted between 1818 and 1830 were discharged as "recovered," "much improved," or "improved." Similarly, 60 percent of the 1,841 patients admitted at Bloomingdale Asylum in New York between 1821 and 1844 were discharged either as "cured" or "improved." Friends Asylum in Philadelphia regularly reported that approximately 50 percent of all admissions left cured. Even the state hospitals initially reported good outcomes During Worcester State Lunatic Asylum's first seven years, more than 80 percent of those who had been ill for less than a year prior to admission "recovered," which meant that they could return to their families and be expected to function at an acceptable level.[27]

In spite of these outstanding results, by the end of the 19th century, conditions in most hospitals were no longer conducive to moral treatment, and practitioners who worked with the mentally ill became utterly pessimistic in their hope for patient recovery. This pessimism set the scene for the emergence of applied eugenics in the early 20th century.[28]

Whitaker persuasively argues that the downfall of moral treatment was caused, in part, by the bureaucratic intrusion of professional medicine.[29] Whitaker's analysis is similar to Ivan Illich's argument that professionalization and bureaucratization of a field, such as medicine or education, can result in "paradoxical counterproductivty," in which the field begins to produce the exact opposite of its stated intent.[30] Whitaker believes that the profession of psychiatry, envious of the success of moral therapy, engaged in a power grab in which doctors lobbied the government to install policies that required all hospitals to maintain a physician as superintendent. By 1844, superintendents of mental hospitals had formed the Association of Medical Superintendents of American Institutions for the Insane, which became yet another platform to lobby for more control of mental patient treatment by physicians. As physicians took over the asylums, they brought with them a reductive conception of mental illness and a return to inhumane treatments such as restraints, sedatives, and devices of torture.

Moral treatment was also defeated by its own success. The popularity of the approach led to overcrowding in hospitals and, consequently, a lack of resources and unhealthy conditions. Recovery rates began to fall precipitously as more and more patients clamored for attention and care.[31] In a detailed historical analysis of psychiatry between the years 1880 and 1940, Ian Robert Downbiggin builds a case that psychiatrists who were superintendents of mental hospitals in the late 19th century became increasingly demoralized as they were expected to treat more and more patients with fewer and fewer resources, which led to a sense of pessimism about the potential for recovery among the mentally ill.[32] Psychiatrists countered this pessimism with biological explanations for insanity, which in turn led many to gravitate toward eugenic solutions for psychiatric problems.

Thomas Malthus, an English scholar whose ideas were popular in the early 1800s, fomented fear in the general public that humans were likely to overpopulate the earth, and that diseased people would cause a degeneration of the species.[33] In the late 1800s, Darwin's half-cousin Francis Galton, who was deeply influenced by Darwin's theory of natural selection and Malthus's concerns about the human race, was the first to coin the term *eugenics*—selective breeding for the purpose of improving the quality of the human race.[34] Child psychiatry emerged as a field during the height of the eugenics movement in the early 20th century.[35] In this climate, children were assessed, categorized, and treated for deficits of intelligence. In one system of classification, four different categories of *idiot* were delineated: moderate, severe, and profoundly mentally retarded; imbecility with severe defects in social development; backward or feebleminded; and simple or superficial retardation with slow development.[36] Up through the 1850s, children with behavioral problems were housed with adults in mental hospitals, but with the emergence of the culture of eugenics, children began to be segregated and received special services at places such as Great Ormond Street Hospital in London. With policies such as the Elementary Education (Defective and Epileptic Children) Act, established in 1899, children who were thought to have defective genes were segregated from the rest of society. In 1913, England established the Royal Commission on the Care and Control of the Feeble-Minded, which was designed to regulate marriage and control reproduction among those who were deemed unfit. By the mid-1930s, individuals such as William Partlow, superintendent of the Alabama State School for Mental Deficients, were granted the authority to sterilize the feebleminded in their charge.

The eugenics movement was driven by a zenophobic terror of immigrants and migrant workers who were deemed a threat to the white, Anglo-Saxon upper classes as urban areas became increasingly overcrowded and unsanitary. It was funded by the enormous pockets of individuals such as Andrew Carnegie, who supported the research of Charles Davenport at the Eugenics Record Office at Cold Spring Rarbor, Long Island. The funds available to eugenicists enabled the movement to infect academic scholarship, government policy, and public opinion. For example, in 1921, the American Museum of Natural History hosted the Second International Congress on Eugenics, which was funded by the Carnegie Foundation and the Rockefeller Foundation.[37]

In 1926, the American Eugenics Society was founded with a major contribution from Rockefeller. By establishing a zeitgeist in the culture, in which those with mental illness were seen to be genetically defective and a threat to the race, the eugenics movement gradually led to sweeping changes in social policy, such that individuals with mental illness were increasingly segregated and then sterilized through legal procedures. By 1921, 3,233 eugenic sterilizations had been conducted in the United States alone.[38] These sterilization laws were challenged for their constitutionality in the U.S. Supreme Court in the case of *Buck v. Bell*. Sadly, the right of the states to sterilize their own people was upheld. This legal and moral catastrophe set a global precedent that eventually led to the legalization of sterilization in many other countries, including Norway, Sweden, Finland, and Iceland.[39] When Adolf Hitler came to power and established his own program of eugenics, he was empowered by the U.S. Supreme Court decision. Within a decade, the Nazi eugenics project had escalated to the point to which it rationalized the extermination of human beings in gas chambers—a tragic chapter in history we all know too well. With Hitler's final solution, the evils of eugenics were taken to their logical extreme, and it was this realization that led to the retreat of the eugenics movement into relative obscurity.

What lessons can we take from this tragic period of history? First, understanding mental illness as exclusively genetic in origin is highly problematic and not as compelling as an approach that takes into account biological, psychological, and social factors as conceptualized in the "biopsychosocial model."[40] We are quick to assign personal blame (e.g., faulty genes) without consideration of situational and sociocultural factors that are often the cause of psychological disturbance and that color how clinicians and how we as a society perceive that disturbance.[41] When we fall prey to irrational attributions of blame to the biological makeup of individuals, nightmarish consequences, such as the eugenics movement, are apt to result.

Second, when physicians are not given sufficient resources to cope with human suffering, they are more prone to use irrational and pessimistic internal attributions, especially biologically reductive disease mongering that stigmatizes their patients and prevents them from accessing the kind of interventions that they need. When society and psychiatric patients themselves begin to internalize these beliefs, patients are further stigmatized and even less likely to seek out effective care.[42]

The era of moral treatment teaches us that successful treatment of many forms of mental illness requires neither biological explanations nor medical specialty. What seems to have made moral therapy—first practiced by the Quakers with no background in medicine—so successful? Very simply, they applied the age-old belief that tender loving care can go a long way toward healing a person who is suffering from mental anguish. This insight is mirrored by contemporary science on the effectiveness of psychotherapy. A large and growing body of evidence is now telling us that the most important and powerful ingredient in the effective treatment of mental illness is the healing presence of another person who empathizes with and cares about the person who is suffering.[43]

LESSONS FROM HISTORY, PART 2: FREUD AND THE COCAINE FAD

When I introduce the subject of psychoanalysis to my undergraduates, I ask them what they have heard about Sigmund Freud. Invariably, at least one student acknowledges that he or she has heard about his abuse of cocaine and writes him off as a quack. It takes some effort to convince students that in Freud's time, cocaine was not considered to be a harmful narcotic. On the contrary, it appeared to be a miracle drug that was widely prescribed by physicians for any and all ailments.[44] At the height of the Victorian era, cocaine was celebrated by the likes of Thomas Edison, Queen Victoria, and even Pope Leo XIII, according to historian Howard Merkel.[45]

The coca plant was imported from South America to Europe, and drug companies processed it to create a concentrated version, cocaine hydrochloride. This concentrated, powdered form was more potent than chewing on the leaves of the coca plant. The drug companies worked hard to market their product, and physicians were a favorite target of their marketing strategies. Freud and his colleagues were sold on the medicinal potential of the drug, much like physicians today who succumb to the not-so-subtle persuasion of drug marketers.

Freud was so swept up in the promise of cocaine that he published an essay extolling its virtues and conjectured that he would demonstrate that the plant had curative powers exceeding even morphine. He started taking the drug himself and came to believe that it was a cure for his depression.

It did not take long for reality to come crashing down upon Freud. His habit grew steadily, and it is likely that he became addicted. In the meantime, the addictive properties of cocaine and its side effects became publicly known. Within a few years, Coca-Cola removed cocaine from their formula. The cocaine fad fell hard. By 1914, it became illegal to use it for nonmedical purposes as a result of the Harrison Narcotic Act. Freud moved on, but not without the stigma of having endorsed a drug that that was not only ineffective but harmful. Freud's premature embrace of cocaine and exuberant endorsement holds important lessons.

I sometimes imagine students, a century from now, listening to a professor lecture about the rampant and indiscriminate use of psychiatric medications in the 21st century such as antidepressants, psychostimulants, and antipsychotics. Will this appear to them to be as misguided as Freud's cocaine prescriptions? Freud's legacy of cocaine abuse should remind those of us who work in the mental health field, that we should never allow ourselves to fall prey to the kind of self-serving bias that diminishes our critical faculties, even when we are caught up in the exuberant hope and optimism of a potential miracle cure. And, of course, we are reminded that we need to discriminate between marketing hype and real science.

LESSONS FROM HISTORY, PART 3: ICE PICK LOBOTOMIES

Walter Freeman's invention of the lobotomy in 1935 as a cure for mental illness is another tragic moment in the history of psychiatry— one that many of us prefer to forget. El-Hai's biography of Walter Freeman portrays him as a man driven by ambition, who stumbled upon a surgical means of curing his patients who suffered from severe mental illness.[46] Freeman streamlined his surgery until it became a very simple procedure that required little more than an anesthetic, an ice pick, and about 10 minutes of his time. The procedure involved penetrating the eye socket with an ice pick–like instrument and hammering it through the thin shell of skull until it penetrated the brain. Once in the brain, Freeman was able to sever the fibers connecting the frontal lobe to the limbic system in the midbrain. The frontal lobe is associated with executive functioning, and the limbic system is linked to mental activities such as emotional reactions and memory.[47] Severing the means by which these parts of the brain communicate brings an abrupt end to the kinds of rumination and self-focused attention that perpetuate many of the worst forms of mental illness. However, this so-called cure came at a very costly price.

As practitioners and researchers began to discover, patients who received the lobotomy tended to become unmotivated, docile, and dysfunctional in their daily activities.[48] The frontal lobe, as the seat of executive functioning, is responsible for the coordination of goal-related activities. By severing this part of the brain from the motivational center of the limbic system, the person essentially becomes incapable of translating their mental goals into action. Patients become easier to control, but at the considerable cost of severe and permanent disability that renders them incapable of caring for themselves. Despite these findings, many patients eagerly lined up for Freeman, naïve in their benevolent perceptions of the medical doctor and the hope of escaping their mental pain. In his 2002 book *Mad in America*, Whitaker describes how housewives, when learning of the lobotomy procedure in the news, eagerly sought out the procedure, as if it were a new fashionable line of clothing, without realizing the cost.[49] This is not unlike the enthusiasm with which the general public has embraced psychiatric drugs. Walter Freeman's ice pick lobotomies provide us with another lesson: Even when a new treatment seems to work to reduce symptoms, it does not mean that we should immediately embrace it. The side effects can be far more devastating than the symptoms that were the focus of treatment in the first place. A sensible approach is one that carefully measures and balances the potential benefits against the potential risks, always leaning in the direction of caution.

LESSONS FROM HISTORY, PART 4: FROM MESMERISM TO ANTIDEPRESSANTS

Franz Anton Mesmer was a physician of German origin who spent most of his professional career in France during the late 18th century. His theory, known as *Mesmerism*, was wildly popular in Europe. Mesmerism was deduced from the best science of the day: Isaac Newton's theory of gravity. Newton suggested that gravity might be a force operating in the body.[50] Newton coined the term *animal gravitation* to describe what he speculated to be an invisible fluid in the body responsive to gravity, which could in turn have effects on human behavior. Picking up on Newton's suggestion, Mesmer theorized that an invisible magnetic force field operates within and around the human body that can cause various mental disorders until they are realigned. Mesmer named this hypothetical force *animal magnetism*.

To test out his theory of animal magnetism, Mesmer began to apply magnets to patients with a variety of medical and psychiatric problems. He performed his magnetic treatments publicly so as to demonstrate to the community the efficacy of his treatments. Remarkably, the magnetic treatments seemed to be miracle cures. Waving a magnetic wand appeared to be a very quick and painless cure for neurosis. At one point, Mesmer used magnets to anesthetize a patient during a limb amputation surgery. Lo and behold, as implausible as it may seem to us today, the patient was free of pain even as doctors worked feverishly to sever his limb. Many people witnessed Mesmer's miracle cures, and not surprisingly, his treatments became the talk of the town.

A Scottish physician by the name of James Braid was a born skeptic who identified a flaw in Mesmer's theory. While Mesmer had demonstrated successful outcomes as a result of his magnetic cures, he had failed to rule out alternative explanations. Braid began to suspect that the magnetic applications were not likely responsible for the cures; as a hypnotist, he hypothesized that the cure had less to do with the procedures employed by Mesmer than with the patient's belief that these procedures would in fact lead to a cure. To test this hypothesis, Braid performed experimental studies in which the medical application of magnetic versus nonmagnetic rods could be compared. Braid discovered that the treatments were successful in both conditions—in other words, the treatment seemed to cure the patient whether or not a magnetic force had actually been applied. Braid concluded that the success of the treatment was attributable to the patient's faith in the doctor's power to heal.

Braid discovered what we now call the *placebo effect*.[51] A *placebo* is a bogus medical procedure, in which a pill or treatment is delivered to a patient in the absence of the curative agent. For example, a patient may be told that they are to receive a pill to reduce hypertension, when in fact they receive a sugar pill. Thousands of research studies have demonstrated the powerful effect of the placebo on a wide variety of medical problems. For example, in the treatment of irritable bowel syndrome, placebo effects account for a 40 percent decrease in symptoms.[52]

Today, it is widely understood that before a medical treatment is considered to be valid, it should be submitted to scientific scrutiny in order to rule out placebo effects. The gold-standard scientific procedure for ruling out the placebo effect is the randomized, controlled clinical trial. In this type of experiment, patients are randomly assigned to two or more conditions of the treatment. For example, in a simple research design, one group of participants is randomly selected to receive the treatment, and the remaining participants are given a placebo. The treatment is considered to be effective if the results of the experiment demonstrate that the treatment group improves to a significantly greater extent than the placebo group. In addition, differences between the treatment and placebo groups should not only be *statistically* significant, but also *clinically* significant. That is, the difference should be of sufficient magnitude that it would substantially improve the health and quality of life of the patient. And the benefits of the treatment should clearly outweigh negative side effects. Thanks to James Braid, we can take another lesson from history: the fact that a treatment *appears* to work does not guarantee that the treatment is in fact efficacious unless we rule out the placebo effect.

While we tend to believe that modern medicine routinely relies on rigorous research before introducing new treatments, psychiatry currently has another version of Mesmerism in the guise of antidepressant medication designed to cure chemical imbalances. Psychologist Irving Kirsh has garnered powerful and compelling empirical evidence that antidepressant medication is no better than placebo.[53] Kirsch and his colleagues have gathered data on clinical trials of antidepressants that were submitted by drug companies to the FDA in order to gain approval for use in the treatment of depression. Using advanced statistical methods of meta-analysis, they found that while antidepressants demonstrated a slight improvement over placebo, this improvement was so small as to be clinically insignificant. Moreover, any difference between the antidepressant groups and the placebo groups could be better accounted for as a result of side effects of the antidepressants, which alerted the treatment group to the fact that they were receiving the active treatment rather than the placebo. When side effect–inducing active placebos are used instead, the difference between antidepressants and placebos seems to disappear. Should anyone question the integrity of Kirsch's research, his findings on antidepressants have been successfully replicated by other researchers.[54]

Kirsch has also exposed the chemical imbalance theory of depression to be an unproven psychiatric myth.[55] No evidence has ever been found to substantiate the claim that people who are depressed have a chemical imbalance. Research has been done in which serotonin and norepinephrine were experimentally reduced in healthy research participants, which in theory should have caused depression. It did not. Also, a drug called trianeptine has been shown to be as effective as the SSRI antidepressants, which elevate levels of seretonin in the brain. And yet, traneptine *enhances* reuptake of serotonin, the exact opposite chemical action of the antidepressants. If the chemical imbalance theory were correct, trianeptine would worsen depression, not improve it. These findings and others, as reviewed by Kirsch, demonstrate that the chemical imbalance theory is merely a story used by drug companies to market a product and employed by physicians to compel their patients to take medication. The evidence overwhelmingly leads to the conclusion that the chemical imbalance theory is a myth destined to join Mesmerism on the junk heap of discarded ideas of science and medicine.

Kirsch's exposure of the myth of antidepressants is consistent with Braid's debunking of the myth of Mesmerism. Like Mesmer's theory of animal magnetism and his treatment with magnets, antidepressants are an enormously popular and even faddish treatment for depression. Mesmer's theory drew inspiration from advances in Newton's scientific breakthrough. Similarly, the chemical imbalance theory of depression, while a myth, modeled itself on important advances in neuroscience. The appeal to new and well-established scientific fact gives power to the illusion of the chemical imbalance in depression and its alleged chemical cure in the form of SSRI antidepressants. The revelation that depression is not caused by a chemical imbalance could be the start of a domino effect in psychiatric treatment because genetically influenced chemical imbalances have been promoted as the root of a majority of psychiatric disturbances including schizophrenia, bipolar disorder, and anxiety to name a few.

The exposure of the antidepressant myth was a blow to modern psychiatry (although the marketing machine of the pharmaceutical giants has so far managed to keep the myth alive). But if that was not enough, in the same year, psychiatry also saw the publication of several other very persuasive books warning about the dangers of current psychiatric practice. In a June 2011 issue of the *New York Review of Books,* Marcia Angell, former editor of the *New England Journal of Medicine,* reviewed these texts in a bombshell essay that is still reverberating through the psychiatric community.[56] In addition to Kirsch's book, *The Emperor's New Drugs: Exploding the Antidepressant Myth,* Angell also reviewed Robert Whitaker's *Anatomy of an Epidemic: Magic Bullets, Psychiatric Drugs, and the Astonishing Rise of Mental Illness in America* and Daniel Carlat's *Unhinged: The Trouble with Psychiatry—A Doctor's Revelations About a Profession in Crisis.*[57] All three books offer a powerful, persuasive, and scientifically valid critique of contemporary psychiatry by credible sources. The impact of Angell's article is evident by an article in *Forbes* magazine featured in the July 2011 issue instructing investors that, "among the public, scholars, and within the medical profession, a backlash has developed against the widespread use of psychoactive drugs"[58]—a warning to Wall Street that it may be time to retreat from investments in psychopharmacology.

Whereas Kirsch has exposed antidepressants as being *no better* than placebo, Robert Whitaker's examination of the long-term effects of psychoactive drugs concludes that psychoactive substances are *far worse* than placebo because in many cases they *cause* long-term disability rather than cure or prevent it. In his book *Anatomy of an Epidemic,* Whitaker examined the long-term impact of a wide range of psychiatric drugs. In the case of antipsychotics, Whitaker concludes that while there is weak evidence of short-term benefits for psychotic patients, there is no evidence that antipsychotics improve long-term outcomes for patients diagnosed with schizophrenia.[59] On the contrary, the available research, beginning with the very earliest studies by the NIMH, reveals that antipsychotic drugs cause deterioration in functioning over the long-term, compared to those who are left untreated with drugs. As Whitaker describes in chapter 1, the long-term use of antipsychotics in children causes permanent damage to the brain and body.

Given what Kirsch and Whitaker reveal about the ineffectual and often dangerous effects of psychotropic medication such as antipsychotics, why has psychiatry continued to treat patients with them? An important factor is that the pharmaceutical industry is obscenely profitable and powerful as Gwen Olsen's compelling analysis reveals in chapter 4.

THE EPIDEMIC OF CHILDREN'S PSYCHIATRIC DISORDERS

How can our history lessons inform our understanding of the epidemic of childhood psychiatric disorders and the increasing reliance on powerful drug treatments such as anitipsychotics? The psychiatric drugging of children is occurring against the backdrop of an enormous economic machine, which Olsen depicts in chapter 4.

One avenue through which Big Pharma holds sway over the practice of psychiatry is through its financial ties to the Task Force of the American Psychiatry Association's *Diagnostic and Statistical Manual of Mental Disorders (DSM).*[60] The *DSM* has been universally adopted by American psychiatrists to diagnose and code their patients' disorders. Investigations by Lisa Cosgrove and colleagues have found that 56 percent of *DSM-IV* task force members had financial ties to the pharmaceutical industry, which represents an egregious conflict of interest.[61] Members on panels for diagnostic categories most relevant to Pharma interests tended to have the most members with Pharma ties: 100 percent of mood disorder panel members, 100 percent of schizophrenia and other psychotic disorders panel members, and 81 percent of anxiety disorder panel members. A new edition of the *DSM* is scheduled to appear in May 2013. The *DSM-5* task force—which is tasked with decisions about which existing diagnoses should be modified or eliminated and which new diagnoses to include—has not only failed to rectify these conflicts of interest, it has seen a 14 percent *increase* in financial links to Pharma among its members.[62] We can witness the power of these influences in the new diagnostic categories for children that are being peddled by the *DSM* task force in preparation for the new *DSM-5* manual.

Two new childhood diagnoses have been proposed for inclusion in the *DSM-5* that increase the risk that children will be treated with atypical antipsychotic drugs. These two diagnostic categories are disruptive mood dysregulation disorder (DMDD) and attenuated psychotic symptoms syndrome (APSS).[63] DMDD is actually a euphemism for PBD, which has become a very controversial diagnosis. Over the past two decades, two American research laboratories were deeply invested in the idea of a PBD—one led by Barbara Geller at Washington University and another by Joseph Biederman at Harvard University. In March of 2009, Joseph Biederman—who at the time was considered to be one of the most respected and powerful researchers in the field of child psychiatry—was exposed for having accepted substantial under-the-table kickbacks from pharmaceutical giant Johnson & Johnson. He was given this money in exchange for promising significant drug sales of their atypical antipsychotic Zyprexa by promoting the drug as a cure for PBD, which he almost single-handedly turned into a popular diagnosis. Fortunately, Biederman was publicly shamed for this egregious violation of scientific ethics.

When Biederman's Faustian bargain with Johnson & Johnson was exposed, the *DSM-5* task force withdrew PBD from consideration. They did something very underhanded and cynical instead: they simply changed the name to DMDD. DMDD has exactly the same diagnostic criteria as Biederman's PBD. And like PBD, it doesn't take a genius to predict this DMDD diagnosis will serve industry well by operating as a means for Pharma to encourage doctors to treat it with atypical antipsychotics.

The chair of the *DSM-IV* task force, Allen Frances, has voiced strong opposition to the DMDD diagnosis.[64] He believes that research on DMDD lacks systematic, empirical research support and would likely serve to pathologize relatively normal children. With regard to the likely treatment approaches to DMDD, Frances writes:

Unfortunately, it is inevitable that this will often consist of atypical antipsychotic drugs because these are heavily marketed and may be helpful in reducing some forms of explosive temper outburst. But their beneficial effects in some must be balanced against their very great dangers when widely used for the many. These medications often cause enormous and rapid weight gains, increasing the risk of diabetes, medical complications, and reduced life span. Their use in severely disturbed kids raises its own set of serious clinical and ethical questions, but it can be justified in extremely exigent circumstance. Their use in kids who are having disturbing (but essentially "normal") developmental or situational storms or are irritable for other reasons (e.g., substance abuse, ADD) would be disastrous—but it will happen and probably often.

The proposal for APSS is perhaps even more insidious than DMDD. Previously known as psychotic risk syndrome, the diagnostic criteria is quite loose and could be used to pathologize normal, gifted, or creative children who may be eccentric but worry their anxious parents and overwhelm their overworked teachers and physicians. These harried professionals who may have limited expertise in child development may readily confuse imaginative behavior and magical thinking that is part and parcel of childhood with psychosis. Research on the detection and treatment of psychosis in childhood is so limited as to be almost nonexistent, and its inclusion in the *DSM-5* will almost surely mean that many children will receive a false-positive diagnosis and the stigma that goes along with it, not to mention the side effects and risk of long-term disability associated with a treatment regime of toxic atypical antipsychotic drugs.[65] Allen Frances has spoken out against the APSS diagnosis as well and estimates that the diagnosis would lead to a false diagnosis rate of 70–90 percent at clinics and in general practice.[66] He also recognizes that Big Pharma will exploit this diagnosis to expand the market of atypical antipsychotics into previously unbreached populations of children and adolescents. The use of such medications, says Frances, would be a "prescription for an iatrogenic public health disaster."

CONCLUSIONS

History has taught us that most of what passes for mental illness does not have clear biological causes. Therefore, we must pay attention to the social, cultural, and economic forces at work that create and perpetuate human suffering.[67] History has also shown that pharmaceutical giants have the power and means to invent disorders in order to expand their market share. With the onset of managed care, psychiatrists have been faced with significantly less compensation and time for patients, as well as escalating costs of medical education and malpractice insurance. When mental health professionals lack essential resources, they gravitate to reductive, biological explanations of human suffering that narrow treatment to symptom checklists and drug prescriptions. These impoverished practices disproportionately harm the weakest and most vulnerable. We see this happening to poor and foster care children who are routinely labeled and stigmatized with psychiatric diagnoses and then heavily medicated on polypharmaceutical cocktails that increasingly include antipsychotics.

The fact that atypical antipsychotics are readily available and sometimes quell symptoms in the short run are not sufficient justification for their use. All treatment approaches, especially those involving children using powerful drugs must be vetted and empirically proved to be superior to a placebo. We also must identify potential short-term and long-term side effects and carefully weigh the risk of side effects against any potential benefit. Whitaker's comprehensive review of the research on children's treatment with antipsychotics (chapter 1) leaves no doubt that their potential to do harm far outweighs their benefits. In light of this, it is hard to justify their use with children when tried and true psychotherapeutic approaches are readily available. In addition, there is much that parents and the community can do strengthen and protect children's development.

In order for psychiatrists and indeed all mental health practitioners to fulfill their promise to "do no harm," they need to set aside self-serving interests to protect their profession and take the time to listen to and understand the complex psychological and social conditions with which their patients are struggling. It can take heroic efforts to withstand the pressures of one's peers and the temptations of economic gain. But until we do, the epidemic of childhood psychiatric diagnoses and drugging will continue until childhood as we know it will be lost to us forever.

3

Drugging Our Children: A Culture That Has Lost Its Compass

Sharna Olfman

In the wake of World War II, when racism led to the systematic slaughter of millions of Jews and other minorities across Europe, many progressive thinkers embraced a worldview called *cultural relativism* in which all human cultures were deemed to be of equal value. At that time, cultural relativism was widely perceived as an antidote to racism. It encouraged a deeper appreciation of the wisdom, spirituality, and artistry of diverse cultures, some of which had been dismissed or disparaged by Western intellectuals as primitive and inferior because of their lack of technological sophistication. While individual and cultural diversity is a defining feature of our humanity, we are not endlessly malleable: we all share basic psychological and physical needs that must be met to ensure healthy development. In light of the recent and astonishing rise in the number of American children who are being diagnosed with serious psychiatric disorders and treated with antipsychotics and multiple drug regimens, it is legitimate to question whether American culture is meeting those needs.

When we compare the fortunes of American children to those living in countries ravaged by poverty, war, disease, and famine, some people might argue that it is self-indulgent to question whether American society is providing children with what they need for optimal development. After all, they have so much—perhaps too much, in some

Parts of this chapter have appeared elsewhere in the Childhood in America series.

respects. But this argument fails to take two important facts into account. First, the wealth of this nation is not equitably distributed, and the economic gap between the haves and the have-nots is growing apace. Twenty-one percent of all children in the United States live in poverty, and this number rises to 34 percent for African-American and Hispanic children and 50 percent among children of single mothers.[1] These deepening disparities are reflected in a two-tiered system of public education that serves children in poor and wealthy neighborhoods very differently, and in the increasing violence and despair in inner-city neighborhoods. Second, once our essential needs for food and safety are met, economic prosperity is not correlated with psychological well-being.[2] As I documented in a previous book, *Childhood Lost*,[3] children in the United States at *all* income levels are being challenged by a variety of environmental assaults that undermine healthy physical and psychological development. As a consequence, many American children are being taxed beyond their capacity for healthy adaptation, and parenting has become intolerably labor intensive.

At this critical juncture, it is imperative that we identify children's essential needs, needs that all cultures must meet to ensure that they reach their full human potential. Globalization makes the project of understanding what it means to be human all the more urgent. As technologies enable ever more rapid international communication and travel, the earth is being rapidly transformed into a global village with an increasingly homogenous culture. However, this new global culture is created and defined by corporations whose values and goals are promoted efficiently and relentlessly around the world by powerful media conglomerates. But corporate culture is indifferent at best, and hostile at worst, to the world's children, and it is killing our planet. And so, while preserving the richness of local cultures, we must strive to create an overarching, "child honoring"[4] sensibility— one that is defined *not* by corporate interests that serve the elite, but by humane consideration of children's universal human needs.

THE BUILDING BLOCKS OF CHILDREN'S MENTAL HEALTH: CARE AND COMMUNITY

Urie Bronfenbrenner, one of the leading scholars in developmental psychology, found it sobering to discover that after 50 years of work in the field, he was able to distill the necessary conditions for healthy child development down to two facts. In order to become fully intact human beings, he concluded, children need:

- "The enduring, irrational involvement of one or more adults . . . [i]n short, *somebody has to be crazy about that kid.*"

- And caregivers in turn "need public policies and practices that provide opportunity, status, resources, encouragement, stability, example, and above all *time* for parenthood."[5]

To express it even more simply, children need unconditional love and consistent care from their families, and families in turn need a village to support their efforts. These two principles not only capture the essence of Bronfenbrenner's prolific research, but also that of a number of towering figures in child psychology. In recent years, with the advent of brain imaging techniques, researcher Allan Schore and his colleagues have documented that reliable, loving care during infancy and early childhood has a profound impact on the development of regions of the brain that are critical for regulating emotions and coping with stress. And the ability to regulate feelings and manage stress is the hallmark of mental health.[6]

In this section, I describe the kind of care and community support that all children need, and some of the adverse consequences for children's mental health when these needs are not met, as is increasingly the case in the United States. In so doing, I contest the prevailing belief that psychological disturbances in childhood are predominantly the result of genetically primed brain disorders. When brain disorders are in fact implicated, research suggests that neglect or trauma in early childhood are more likely the causal factors. Instead, I emphasize the role of family and culture in fostering children's mental health.

A few generations ago, new parents expected to learn how to parent their children effectively from their own parents, and from hands-on experience gleaned from helping to care for younger siblings and cousins in stable family and community networks. But in recent decades, technological innovation and globalization have engendered radical changes in our lifestyles, and as a result, the lessons to be learned from our parents and grandparents may seem obsolete. In addition, changes in the workplace require many adults to relocate frequently, separating young parents from their families of origin. And so, new parents must often sort out the challenges and complexities of parenthood for themselves.

A PORTRAIT OF CARE

Time and again over the past half century, researchers have demonstrated that a relationship with at least one loving, responsive, and dependable caregiver is essential for a child's well-being. The quality of this relationship extends well beyond the mere provision of food and shelter and shapes intellectual, language, personality, social, emotional, and brain development. This caregiver-infant relationship is called "attachment."[7] It is not essential that the caregiver in the attachment relationship be the biological mother. Any adult who—in Bronfenbrenners's inimitable words—is "crazy about that kid" can serve as an attachment figure, and in fact, it is better for the child to have more than one caregiver to rely on.

As psychologist Robert Karen explains in *Becoming Attached*:

The concept of "attachment," born in British psychoanalysis some forty years ago and nurtured to near maturity in the developmental psychology departments of American universities . . . encompasses both the quality and strength of the parent-child bond, the ways in which it forms and develops, how it can be damaged and repaired, and the long-term impact of separations, losses, wounds, and deprivations. Beyond that, *it is a theory of love and its central place in human life.*[8]

Attachment—An Anthropological Perspective

Beyond the immediate pleasure that tender, loving care might give an infant or young child, why does its presence or absence have profound psychological consequences that reverberate throughout our lives? In *Childhood Lost*, anthropologist Meredith Small helps us to understand why the attachment between parent and child is of such central importance. Small explains,

Humans, like all primates, are designed to be involved with the upbringing of their offspring for many years, but as we will see, particular evolutionary pressures have rendered the human caregiver-child relationship especially intense and long-lasting. About four million years ago . . . when early humans stood up and started to walk on two legs, that type of locomotion required an increase in the gluteus maximus and minimus muscles which in turn pushed for a short and broad bony pelvic shape. As a result, the pelvic opening, or birth canal, also changed; the opening became essential ovoid instead of round with the sacrum tilted inward forming a bowl. This change in pelvic architecture was not a problem at first because our earliest ancestors still had small brains—comparable in size to the brains of modern chimpanzees—and infants could easily navigate the birth canal. The real crisis came about 1.5 million years ago when there was intense pressure for brain growth in the human lineage and suddenly babies had much bigger heads relative to the size of the pelvic opening. At this point, evolution had to make a compromise because there is only so far you can push the width of the pelvis to accommodate infant head size; if the human pelvis were any wider, women would not be able to walk.

Instead, Natural Selection opted for another route; human infants are born too soon—neurologically unfinished compared to other primates. As a result they are physically and emotionally very dependent. But this level of dependence could not have appeared if there hadn't been some corresponding evolutionary shift in parental behavior that facilitated the capacity to respond to infant needs. And so, there must have been a "co-evolution" of dependent infants and responding adults for human infants to have survived. A human newborn, therefore, is designed by evolution to be "entwined" with an adult of its species. In other words, human infants have evolved to be "attached" both emotionally and physically to their caregivers and when that attachment is denied, the infant is at risk.[9]

Small also reminds us that for 95 percent of our human history, we were all hunter-gatherers. And it was in this physical and social milieu that our species evolved. And so, studying the few extant hunter-gatherer tribes provides us with a window on the conditions in which we first evolved as a species and the way that we are designed to live and raise our children. Today, most people on earth practice a subsistence form of farming called small plot horticulture, and so it is instructive to examine the parenting practices of these societies as well. Why? Because in spite of the headlong pace of technological change, which repeatedly reshapes our social, cultural, and economic lives, children's irreducible needs endure. Therefore, parents cannot simply adjust themselves and their children to prevailing conditions. They must also seek to adjust conditions to address their—and their children's—real human needs.

A survey of different hunter-gatherer and horticultural groups reveals the rich diversity of beliefs, values, and lifestyles that is typical of our species. But despite these variations, a common pattern emerges—in the preindustrial milieu, infants are in almost constant skin contact with their caregivers, who respond immediately to their needs and never leave them to cry. This style of infant care is not just an artifact of poverty or ignorance. It is also standard practice in technologically advanced countries like Japan. In fact, even today, it is typical of the vast majority of human societies. And this style of care is precisely what a half century of attachment research tells us that infants need for optimal psychological and neurological development.

The Premature Push for Independence

It is striking that the United States—where so much attachment research is conducted—is one of the few countries in which parents do not routinely care for their infants in these physically responsive ways that are optimal for psychological and neurological development. Why is this so? As Small suggests,

The primary goal of Western—that is North American and European parents, but especially American parents—is independence and self-reliance for children. This push for independence is most striking in infancy when babies are expected to sleep alone and are fed on a schedule. Western parents also expect infants to "self comfort" when they cry so many parents delay responses to crying or do not respond at all but believe in a policy of letting the infant "cry it out."

This caretaking style results in many hours during which infants are not held and are not part of a social group. Western babies are held 50% less than in all other cultures, spend 60% of day time alone, and the West is the only culture in which babies are expected to sleep alone.[10]

Paradoxically though, infants who are in constant physical contact with their caregivers and never left to cry—as opposed to infants who are trained to be independent by being left alone—are much more likely to become confident, independent children. When left for hours to cry herself to sleep, day after day, week after week, an infant will eventually stop crying and become well behaved. But inwardly, she may be paralyzed with fear, seething with anger, or overwhelmed with sadness. And in the process, she is acquiring an overarching orientation of mistrust—of herself, of others, of her world. While learning to self-comfort and not to cry, other important lessons are being learned as well: that her needs and feelings are insignificant, that she can't rely on others to help her when she is in pain, that how she feels is not particularly informative, and that how she communicates is not particularly effective. By contrast, the infant who is in continual contact with her caregivers, who take seriously and respond quickly to her needs as they arise, builds up an image of herself as competent, of her family as loving, and of her world as safe. And it is this infant who will acquire the confidence with which to exercise true independence.

The Dance of Attachment

Given how vital attachment is to the infant's survival, it should not come as a surprise that human infants are born with a number of characteristics and instinctive behaviors that help to woo the parent into a loving relationship. Research has shown that infants' physical characteristics—their round faces and eyes, soft skin, gentle grasp, the way they mold their bodies when held, radiant smiles, and coos and babbles—are deeply appealing to adults. In addition, from birth, infants are attracted to the smell of their mothers' breast milk, the sound of her voice, the rhythm of her heart beat, the touch of her skin.[11] Daniel Stern's analysis of videos of infants and mothers revealed that quite unconsciously, they engage in a synchronous dance as first one and then the other gaze, touch, and communicate with each other verbally and nonverbally.[12] Infants are so attuned to and dependent on this dance of attachment that they become distressed when a beloved caregiver does not return their smile. Touch is a key element in the attachment relationship. Research has shown that when premature infants are held and stroked each day, they show more rapid neural and physical development than those who receive standard hospital care.[13]

Born Too Soon

Because babies are born too soon—neurologically unfinished—during the first several months of life, human infants are not yet capable of regulating their bodies. Therefore, the attachment or entwined relationship is one of physiological and not just emotional dependency. Sleep expert James McKenna has demonstrated that when nursing mothers and their infants share sleep, their heart rates, brain waves, breathing patterns, and sleep cycles become synchronized.[14]

Breast-feeding also helps to regulate and augment their physiological processes. Over and above the nourishing proteins, minerals, vitamins, fats and sugars, breast milk also supplies antibodies to assist the infant's immature immune system, growth factors that help in tissue development and maturation, and a variety of hormones, neuropeptides, and natural opioids that subtly shape brain development and behavior. The breast has been described as the "external counterpart of the placenta, picking up where [it] left off the task of ushering the infant toward physical and neurological completion."[15]

Learning to Feel

The attachment relationship helps infants to modulate, interpret, and communicate emotions. Sue Gerhardt describes this process in *Why Love Matters: How Affection Shapes a Baby's Brain:*

To become fully human, the baby's basic responses need to be elaborated and developed into more specific and complex feelings. With parental guidance, the basic state of "feeling bad" can get differentiated into a range of feelings like irritation, disappointment, anger, annoyance and hurt. Again, the baby or toddler can't make these distinctions without help from those in the know. The parent must also help the baby to become aware of his own feelings and this is done by holding up a virtual mirror to the baby, talking in baby talk and emphasizing and exaggerating words and gestures so that the baby can realize that this is not mum or dad just expressing themselves, this is them "showing" me my feelings. It is a kind of "psychofeedback" which provides the introduction to a human culture in which we can interpret both our own and others' feelings and thoughts. Parents bring the baby into this more sophisticated emotional world by identifying feelings and labeling them clearly. Usually this teaching happens quite unselfconsciously.[16]

Brain Development

In recent years, with the help of brain-imaging technologies, Allan Schore and his colleagues at the UCLA school of medicine have documented that brain development in the first few years of life is dependent on the social and sensory stimulation that is part and parcel of the attachment relationship.[17] Despite a growth industry in flash cards, videos, toys, and software, which boasts that it can turn your baby into the next Einstein, it is human rather than electronic stimulation that grows a baby's brain. The human touch, voice, gaze, and smile trigger a complex cascade of neurochemicals that catalyze growth in regions of the brain that play a critical role in our ability to empathize, control our impulses, and develop a sense of self. One of the most vital brain regions to develop as an outgrowth of attachment relationships is the orbitofrontal cortex.

The orbitofrontal cortex plays a key role in emotional life. It enables us to empathize with others and to control our emotional responses. Although social emotions, such as the pain of separation from a loved one and shame, originate in the amygdala and hypothalamus, the orbitofrontal cortex serves to control our impulses and help us express ourselves in socially appropriate and reflective ways. It is very significant that the prefrontal cortex and the orbitofrontal cortex have a growth spurt between 6 and 12 months of age, corresponding exactly with when the attachment bond is being consolidated. There is a second growth spurt in early toddlerhood, around the time the child begins to walk—which is also a period of intense pleasure between parent and child.[18]

In a study conducted with Romanian orphans who had no opportunity to form attachments with caregivers during infancy and early childhood, brain imaging revealed a black hole where the orbitofrontal cortex should be. People who sustain damage to the orbitofrontal cortex become insensitive to social and emotional cues. They may also be prone to dissociation or even to sociopathy.[19]

After the orbitofrontal cortex has matured, other areas of the social-emotional brain begin to mature including the anterior cingulate, which helps us to tune into our feelings. Soon thereafter, the dorsolateral prefrontal cortex—the primary site of working memory—begins to develop. Together, the anterior cingulate and dorsolateral cortex facilitate verbal and nonverbal communication of feelings. During the third year of life, the hippocampus, which plays a key role in long-term memory, begins to mature and becomes strongly linked to the anterior cingulate and the dorsolateral prefrontal cortex. The hippocampus enables the child to create a personal narrative with a past and a future, and so, for the first time, she has an enduring sense of self and no longer lives just in the moment. This sequence of postnatal brain development is largely dependent on the sensory, intellectual, and emotional stimulation that is integral to the attachment relationship.[20]

Beyond Attachment

The style of parenting that fosters attachment is ideal during infancy and early toddlerhood. But what then? Although space constraints prevent me from exploring their work at length, the parenting research of Diana Baumrind and Erik Erikson's psychosocial theory of development provide excellent guidelines beyond the intense early months of attachment parenting.

Authoritative Parenting

In the 1970s, Baumrind conducted research to discern what style of parenting is optimal for psychological development. She discovered that an approach to parenting that she named *authoritative* has the best long-term outcomes for children. In the decades that have ensued, her research has been replicated and elaborated, and there is now wide consensus among parenting experts that this approach fosters healthy development.[21]

Authoritative parents are warm, attentive, and sensitive to their children's needs. At the same time, they consistently assert age-appropriate expectations and responsibilities. So for example, their young children know that they are not to eat cookies before dinner and that they must do their homework, complete household tasks, and treat others with respect. When making their expectations known, these parents provide their children with a cogent rationale. As a result, over time, their children internalize their parents' underlying motives and values, so that they don't remain dependent on authority figures to do the right thing. As children get older, authoritative parents grant their children increasing autonomy over decisions that affect them, thereby gently ushering them along their journey toward adulthood.

Authoritative parenting has been linked to a variety of positive outcomes. During the preschool years, children of authoritative parents are happier, have better impulse control, persevere at challenging tasks, and are more cooperative at school. Older children have higher self-esteem, are more socially and morally mature, and perform better at school.[22]

Psychosocial Stages

Psychoanalyst Erik Erikson's theory of psychosocial development describes the central psychological challenges that confront all human beings at different stages of the life cycle.[23] The central psychological challenge of infancy is the acquisition of *trust*. Securely attached infants whose caregivers consistently respond to their needs in a loving and timely fashion come to approach life with optimism. Children who are imbued with trust find it easier to acquire *autonomy* in toddlerhood. Toddlers have a burgeoning sense of self that is ushered in by an explosion of new intellectual, linguistic, and motor skills. Suddenly, they are walking, talking, climbing, and exploring. Parents who allow their toddlers to do for themselves whether it be climbing the stairs, putting on their own shirt, or feeding themselves, without providing absolute freedom (which would be unsafe) or too little freedom (which conveys a message of incompetence), provide optimal support during their bid for autonomy. During the preschool years, children need time for unstructured imaginative play in natural settings in order to develop *initiative*. Psychologically healthy school-age children feel a natural desire to develop the capacity for *industry*. When children find their passion, whether it be tennis, literature, or woodwork, they will work with great diligence toward mastery when parents and teachers facilitate their efforts as mentors and guides.

The predominant psychological challenge of adolescence is to acquire a coherent and meaningful sense of *identity*. Adolescents who begin their search for identity with a healthy sense of trust, autonomy, initiative, and industry are greatly advantaged. And when they enter adulthood knowing who they are, what they believe in and value, and where they are going in life, they are more capable of achieving the central tasks of adulthood: the capacity for enduring *intimacy* and *generativity*. Generativity refers to our desire to nurture the next generation. While parents and helping professionals such as teachers and therapists may nurture children in direct ways, everyone, whether they be artists, managers, environmentalists, or politicians, can make generative choices that inspire or secure the safety and prospects of the next generation.

And now we come full circle. Adults who were securely attached infants with authoritative parents who helped them to successfully negotiate the central psychological challenges of childhood will acquire a healthy sense of identity, which is a precursor for intimacy and generativity. The capacity to sustain intimacy and act generatively are in turn necessary to successfully parent one's own children. In other words, adults who lack trust, autonomy, initiative, industry, and a strong sense of identity will be greatly compromised in their ability to offer intimate and altruistic care to their children.

PORTRAIT OF COMMUNITY

As anthropologist Meredith Small reminds us, there is an evolutionary push toward an entwined or attachment relationship with our children that is as old as our primate history. But our potential for intimacy and generativity will not be actualized unless we ourselves have been the recipients of responsive and responsible care from our own parents. Harlow's research with monkeys revealed that infant monkeys who were separated from their mothers at birth were incapable of nurturing their own offspring.[24] But even when we were well parented ourselves, our innate predisposition to parent must be augmented by direct experience with caregiving, as well as a healthy dose of intelligence and energy. And still these circumstances do not suffice. In Bronfenbrenner's evocative words: "The heart of our social system is the family. If we are to maintain the health of our society, we must discover the best means of nurturing that heart."[25] In other words, parents do not live in a vacuum; the experiences and environments that they (consciously or unwittingly) provide for their children, and protect them from, reflect values and beliefs that have been shaped by their culture. During the first years of life, parents are the conduits of their culture, which is mirrored in the identities their children acquire, and ultimately, in the ways in which they will parent their own children. But cultures also entail systems of governance, education, economy, and overarching values that may support or undermine parents' efforts to nurture their children's development. At present, American culture is failing to support parents' efforts to raise their children. This is due to the fact that public policies in support of families are woefully lacking and significantly inferior to those in all other wealthy nations. As a result, American families are burdened by

- inadequate parental leave and nonexistent child sick leave
- a mental health system that dispenses antipsychotics and polypharmacy as treatments of choice rather than last resort to address children's emotional and behavioral disturbances
- a minimum wage that is not a living wage
- welfare-to-work policies that require thousands of mothers to return to 40-hour work weeks but fail to provide them with affordable, regulated, high-quality child care options
- a two-tiered public education system that delivers inferior education to poor children and frequently ignores individual differences in learning styles and talents

- entertainment and gaming industries that have been given the mandate to police themselves, exposing children to graphic depictions of sex and violence and undermining parental authority and values
- an unregulated advertising industry that spends more than $15 billion annually in direct marketing to children, shaping lifetime addictions to junk food, alcohol, and cigarettes and contributing to a childhood obesity epidemic that is poised to become the leading cause of death in the United States
- weak environmental protection policies that have allowed tens of thousands of toxins to erode our air, soil, and water, undermining children's physical, neurological, and endocrinological development

Why have we not created such policies? Part of the answer lies in the beliefs and values that undergird our culture. First, Americans have a deep faith in and fascination with technologies that remove us farther and farther from the natural world and the constraints of our bodies—even as they destroy our ecosystems and undermine our physical and mental health. So enamored are we of our machines that the information-processing model of thinking, with the computer as its guiding metaphor, has become the backbone of American educational philosophy. Second, Americans give primacy to individual rights and freedoms even when those rights and freedoms undermine humane consideration of our collective responsibilities to children, families, and communities. Our uncritical embrace of technologies and our relentless defense and pursuit of individual goals and pleasures explains

- why we are not deeply alarmed that our kids are interacting with unregulated screen technologies for more hours every day than any other activity but sleep
- why we don't demand that our government ensure that all children have access to high-quality child care
- why we confuse the ability to download and process facts with real education
- why we are so out of touch with children's bedrock human needs for close physical and emotional attachments, fashioned by millions of years of evolution
- why we feel so few qualms about destroying our ecosystem

Our runaway pursuit of individualism leads us to defend the rights of corporate CEOs to pay their workers slave wages, the rights of pornographers to make their websites available to anyone who can turn on a computer, the rights of moviemakers to expose children to graphic acts of violence, and the rights of alcohol and tobacco companies to spawn the next generation of addicts. Tragically, in the process, we have trampled upon our children's fundamental right to grow up in a wholesome environment that supports physical, emotional, and intellectual well-being. Record levels of childhood obesity, asthma, high school failure, psychiatric disturbance, youth suicide, and preteen sex speak to the fact that we are failing our children. The time has come to acknowledge that ensuring a healthy generation of children is not a private matter but a national priority. It is time to temper our pursuit and protection of individual rights when those rights undermine the needs of our youngest citizens.

WHAT PARENTS NEED

If adults are to have the time, resources, and the physical and emotional health necessary to parent their children, they need the following:

- Family, friends, and neighbors who can provide practical and emotional support
- Health care for themselves and their children that is affordable, comprehensive, and not contingent on the whims of an employer
- Affordable housing in safe neighborhoods with amenities that support family life such as parks, community centers, libraries, and grocery stores
- Paid parental and child sick leave that is generous enough to enable parents to form secure attachments with their children and that never obligates them to choose between nursing a sick child or paying the rent
- Day care that is affordable and of the highest quality
- A living wage so that their second shift can be at home with their children
- Flexible work arrangements—that allow them to complete work at home or share a position—without forsaking essential benefits such as health care or permanently compromising opportunities for career advancement
- Public schools that are safe, have small teacher-child ratios, and utilize developmentally sensitive approaches to education
- Media regulation so that their children are no longer relentlessly exposed to violence, pornography, sexism, racism, and commercials for products that undermine their health
- Clean air, soil, and water

American parents who read this wish list may dismiss it as utopian, and yet it describes the status quo in many industrialized nations. In fact, the conditions listed above should be regarded as fundamental human rights because they are the preconditions for fostering attachments and authoritative parenting, which in turn are essential for healthy psychological and neurological development.

WHEN CARE AND COMMUNITY BREAK DOWN

How can a mother who must return to work only days after giving birth—while placing her newborn in substandard care—establish

a secure attachment with her infant? If a single mother must work two
or three low-wage jobs to make ends meet, while her children return
to an empty home, how can she scaffold their arduous journey toward adulthood? And how can she protect them from the tidal wave
of violence, hatred, racism, sexism, and pornography that pervade the
media? And if this mother is the second or third generation to have
raised children under these dangerous and degrading circumstances,
how will she herself acquire the psychological maturity and wisdom
to relate lovingly and responsibly toward her children? But these are
precisely the conditions under which millions of American parents are
obligated to raise their children. As Bronfenbrenner has lamented, "the
comparative lack of family support systems in the United States is so
extreme as to make it unique among modern nations."[26]

Sadly, it appears that support for families in the United States continues to deteriorate in lockstep with the rise in psychiatric disturbances. Psychologist Laura Berk described this downward spiral in
Childhood Lost:

American children and adolescents of all walks of life are experiencing more stress
than their counterparts of the previous generation. An examination of hundreds
of studies of nine-to seventeen-year-old carried out between the 1950s and the
1990s revealed a steady, large increase in anxiety over this period. A combination
of reduced social connectedness and increased environmental dangers (crime, violent media, fear of war, etc.) appeared responsible[.] . . . Interestingly, whereas
societal indicators of diminished social connectedness . . . showed strong associations with children's rising anxiety, economic conditions such as poverty and un-
employment had comparatively little influence. *A child's well-being, it appears, is
less responsive to whether the family has enough money than to whether it promotes close,
supportive bonds with others.* Other changes in the American family also point to a
withering of social connectedness. For example, Americans are less likely to visit
friends, join community organizations, and volunteer in their communities than
they once were. [P]arents and children converse and share leisure time less often
than they did in the past.

Simultaneously, young people's sense of trust in others has weakened. In 1992
only 18.3 percent of high school seniors agreed that one can usually trust people,
compared with 34.5 percent in 1975. Young people's increased anxiety is a natural
response to lower quality relationships. *As social connectedness in the United States
declined, youth suicide rates rose.* Between the 1950s and 1970s, they rose by 300 percent for fifteen—twenty-five-year olds; and between 1980 and 1997, by 109 percent
for ten-to fourteen-year-olds.[27]

CONCLUSION

The galloping breakdown in caregiving and community support is
largely responsible for the epidemic of psychiatric disturbances that
we are now witnessing among America's children. That view is not

very popular, however, because policy-based efforts to heal communities, empower parents, and regulate industry are actively opposed by powerful lobbies for the pharmaceutical, genetic technology, media, education, and food industries. And stellar careers in research are not built upon promoting practices that many of our grandmothers and great-grandmothers knew intuitively to be true. In contrast, the claim that mental health or illness is encoded in our genes is so widespread that social psychologist Carol Travis apparently had no qualms about including the following statement as part of a list of false assumptions that have been "resoundingly disproved by research":

- "The way that parents treat a child in the first five years (three years) (one year) (five minutes) of life is crucial to the child's later intellectual and emotional success."[28]

And this statement was published in the *Chronicle of Higher Education*, one of the most widely read and respected newspapers in academic circles.

Meanwhile, and in spite of all the bipartisan talk about family values, we are not providing even the most rudimentary support to our families, which is what we *must* do if we are to address the root cause of children's psychological disturbances. I close with a quote from Bronfenbrenner:

"One telling criterion of the worth of a society—a criterion that stands the test of history—is the concern of one generation for the next. As we enter our third century, we Americans, compared to other industrialized societies, appear to be abandoning that criterion . . . It would appear that the process of making human beings human is breaking down in American society. To make it work again, we must reweave the unraveling social fabric and revitalize the human bonds essential to sustaining the well-being and development of both present and future generations."[29]

4

The Marketing of Madness and Psychotropic Drugs to Children

Gwen Olsen

The explosion of mental illness diagnoses given to U.S. children in the past 20 years is unprecedented anywhere else in the world. Millions of children have been labeled with childhood mental illnesses and are taking prescribed medications to treat them. The problem is now virtually pandemic in the United States, as an estimated 1 out of 7 school-age children is on at least one psychotropic drug, and many kids are on several. An analysis of the data shows an estimated 40-fold (4,000%) increase in the number of children on psychiatric drugs between 1970 and 2000.[1] Unfortunately, the increased use of these medications has not proved to curb the ensuing mental health crisis. In fact, quite the opposite is occurring. According to U.S. disability figures for mental illness, the daily disability rate of 1,100 people is composed of 850 adults and 250 children, and it is growing.[2]

Since the advent of the psychopharmacological age some 50 years ago with the discovery of Thorazine, there has been no improvement in long-term disability outcomes in mental illness. Yet, the increase in psychotropic drug use continues to eclipse all other drug categories on a year-to-year growth basis and is steadily climbing for children. In 2009, children were by far the largest growth demographic for the pharmaceutical industry, and prescriptions for kids grew at four times the rate of the general population. Over the past 9 years, the most substantial increases in the medicating of children have been seen in conditions not typically associated with kids, such as drugs for type 2 diabetes and antipsychotics.[3] Interestingly, antipsychotic drugs have been shown to cause metabolic dysfunction and induce diabetes, in both children and adults.[4]

These statistics should make us ask the question: If the drugs are not effective in producing improved outcomes for mental health, what is driving the momentum behind this epidemic of drugging our kids? Could it be that the increased awareness created by public service campaigns is driving diagnosis and treatment of these disorders? Or is that merely a component of a much larger marketing initiative on the part of the pharmaceutical industry to expand psychotropic drug use into new patient populations, such as our children?

I spent the span of 15 years in the pharmaceutical industry, learning and employing the most highly effective marketing tactics known in professional sales. My training as a specialist and hospital rep was exceptional, and I was an excellent observer, a good student, and an accomplished participant. So, I can say with some confidence that the pharmaceutical industry has identified a lucrative, new profit center and is pushing expensive, dangerous, antipsychotic drugs on our youngest, most vulnerable citizens—our children. This is exactly how it was done.

DISEASE MONGERING: CREATING FEAR AND ANGST

The problem with the ever-expanding drug market is that there are a finite number of diseases and patients needing treatment. That being said, one of the biggest problems for drug manufacturers is finding new places to expand the usage of existing products that will subsequently gain new indications and patent extensions. That is why a blood pressure drug shown to cause the side effect of hirsutism gets redeveloped and branded into another drug for hair growth and is marketed for baldness.

The pharmaceutical industry is continually on the lookout for expansion markets. Our children are recognized by the pharmaceutical industry to be the most lucrative, long-term expansion market currently available to them. Where kids are concerned, fear created in parents can send them racing to the doctor's office and/or pharmacy in an attempt to protect their children. After all, isn't that what all good parents do?

So, not only is the pharmaceutical industry in the business of selling drugs, it is also in the business of selling fear. In the words of author and health activist Dr. Joseph Mercola, they want you to feel frightened for your health, as that is a very powerful motivating emotion. The goal of the campaign is to create a scenario where relying on them for the solution (to the issue they made you fearful of) is necessary. This creates a dependency and annuity that enriches their bottom line.[5]

Children are a lucrative expansion market for any drug, particularly one that requires lifelong maintenance therapy once initiated. Psychiatric diagnoses are highly subjective and based primarily on third-party interpretation of maladaptive behaviors, rather than medical diagnostic tests such as blood or urine tests, or PET and CAT scans. So increasing psychiatric drug sales is primarily contingent upon increasing the number of psychiatric diagnoses and public awareness of the various diagnoses that will, in turn, result in the expansion of new patient populations to be treated.

The challenge that exists when marketing psychotropic drugs for children is that the pharmaceutical industry cannot market directly to the end consumer. In the case of children, doctors, parents, teachers, counselors, administrators, caretakers, legislators, and so on must be persuaded that these medications are both necessary and beneficial to children. To meet this goal, it is necessary for Pharma to insidiously exert its influence in every aspect of pharmaceutical development, research, reporting, regulation, funding, advertising, promotion, and distribution. And, indeed, they do! The end result is a stealth marketing campaign that can wear many hats and disguises as it manipulates and promotes its self-serving agenda unilaterally throughout the entire health care system.

KEY OPINION LEADERS: PHARMA SHILLS IN ACADEMIA

Unlike disease, which is discovered scientifically in the laboratory by the objective detection of some physical or chemical abnormality, psychiatric illness is subjectively determined by a group of experts from the American Psychiatric Association (APA) who *decide* that certain behaviors (called *symptoms*) are abnormal and then vote these sets of behavior into existence as a disease. For example, attention deficit disorder (ADD) was voted into existence in 1980, and attention deficit/hyperactivity disorder (ADHD) in 1987. No child labeled as ADHD has met a medical standard that confirms the existence of a specific pathology connoting disease. It can't be done because no such standard exists. In the words of retired neurologist Fred Baughman Jr., who has been credited with the discovery of real neurological disease, "ADHD is a total, complete, 100% fraud."[6]

Pediatric bipolar disorder (PBD), another newly developed affliction among American kids, is apparently unique to our area of the world as well. International psychiatrists are perplexed as to why American doctors would so readily buy into this marketing initiative. Prior to the 1990s, scientific literature and clinical experience did not substantiate the existence of a bipolar illness in prepubertal children. However, children and adolescents who are prescribed stimulants such as ADHD medications and antidepressants often suffer manic episodes. So, once these categories of drugs became commonly prescribed to children, bipolar symptoms also became prevalent in pediatric populations. Thus, the literature and physicians began reporting the increased emergence of youth with bipolar symptoms.[7]

A leading child psychiatrist from Harvard affiliated Massachusetts General Hospital in Boston, Joseph Biederman, popularized PBD by providing the diagnostic framework that made it possible. In 1996, Biederman and his colleagues announced that many kids who were previously diagnosed with ADHD were actually bipolar, or were co-morbid for both diseases. Furthermore, he claimed that the condition was much more common than had previously been thought and often appeared when children were only four or five years old.[8] His reconceptualization of children with conduct disorder and ADHD led to a 40-fold increase of bipolar diagnoses in children in the last decade. Biederman's discovery provided Pharma with a new expansion population for what was once an exceedingly rare mental illness (even among adults, the prevalence of bipolar disorder was only estimated to be 1%) and opened up untapped markets for the new atypical antipsychotic drugs, which were competing with older and considerably less expensive generic drugs in the psychiatric market.

Biederman was investigated by Congress for his financial ties to the pharmaceutical industry in 2008, whereupon it was discovered that he had failed to disclose nearly $1.6 million in income from pharmaceutical manufacturers to his Harvard employers. In 2009, Biederman explained the genesis of PBD as such: Since all psychiatric diagnoses "are subjective in children and adults," he said that he and his colleagues had decided that children who presented pronounced behavioral problems should instead be diagnosed with PBD. "These children have been called in the past [as having] conduct disorder, oppositional-defiant disorder. It's not that these children did not exist, they were just under different names," Biederman testified. He went on to say that they had decided that "severe irritability" or "affective storms" would be the determining diagnostic criteria for PBD diagnosis.

Biederman is a prolific psychiatric researcher, whose work is published in prestigious medical journals. In 2007, Dr. Biederman was ranked as the second-highest producer of high-impact papers in the field of psychiatry internationally, with 235 papers cited a total of 7,048 times over the past 10 years as determined by the Institute for

Scientific Information.[9] Furthermore, "Newly disclosed court documents portray Dr. Joseph Biederman . . . as courting drug company money by promising that his work at Massachusetts General Hospital would help promote the use of antipsychotic drugs for youngsters diagnosed with bipolar disorder," which further suggests that the PBD genesis may have been entirely profit driven by corporate interests.[10]

Practically everyone knows of someone's child who has been labeled bipolar. Unfortunately as previously stated, many of these bipolar symptoms stem from prior psychotropic drug use. A large study of children from the Luci Bini Mood Disorders Clinic in New York diagnosed with PBD found that 84 percent of the children treated for bipolar disorder had been previously exposed to psychiatric medications. The study's author reported, "Strikingly, in fewer than 10 percent of the cases was diagnosis of bipolar disorder considered initially."[11] For many years, it had been concluded in the medical literature that mania did not occur in children. The general belief was that manic-depressive states were an illness of the maturing or matured personality only. However, after psychiatrists began prescribing stimulant drugs to hyperactive children in the late 1960s and early 1970s, more and more of these case reports started to emerge in the medical literature.[12]

When I was selling psychiatric drugs, manufacturers of antidepressants recommended that these be used as a diagnostic tool for uncovering latent bipolar illness in depressed patients. It was never suggested to the doctor that the drugs might be the cause of these manic episodes rather than the patient's underlying disease state. Oftentimes, drugs that are administered for ADHD, such as Ritalin and Adderall, as well as SSRI and SNRI antidepressants or even atypical antipsychotics, can induce varying degrees of manic behaviors—including psychosis—as an adverse effect of the drug. These reactions are often unwittingly misdiagnosed by health care providers as symptoms of a *mixed-state* bipolar illness. This form of bipolar illness is considered more severe and generally has a poor prognosis. The symptoms are then exacerbated by the introduction of additional, possibly stronger, cocktails of psychotropic medications to treat the so-called mixed state. Even if a conscientious practitioner later realizes that the child is reacting to a chemical assault on the body and brain and succeeds in detoxifying the child into recovery, the psychiatric labels given early on in life can carry an accompanying stigma that cannot be as easily shaken.

It is unconscionable to think that corporations, much less our doctors, would callously put our children at risk of harm—or even worse, death—for profit, but it is important to understand why many prominent critics of these practices are afraid to speak out. The pharmaceutical industry is just as aggressive in its tactics to silence its critics as it is to woo its supporters. Respected scientists and doctors have been defamed in the press and even fired for daring to draw attention to the hazards and risks of suicide, violence, and premature death associated with the use of psychiatric drugs in children and adolescents.[13]

PUBLISHING FRAUDULENT CLINICAL TESTS, GHOST-WRITTEN JOURNAL ARTICLES, AND TEXTBOOKS

In an attempt to further influence physician prescribing and increase sales, manufacturers often employ ghostwriters to seed the peer-reviewed journals and medical literature with favorable studies and articles regarding their products. Many times, only favorable end points of studies are reviewed, which skews the actual outcomes and clinical significance of the study or data and can entirely spin and misrepresent the information. A huge scandal emerged during the discovery process of the Vioxx lawsuits. Vioxx made blockbuster status in terms of drug sales, until it was removed from the market in 2005 for causing heart attacks in patients. In April 2008, a *Journal of the American Medical Association* (*JAMA*) editorial reported that Merck had drafted a number of research studies for Vioxx and gone doctor shopping to find prestigious physicians to put their names on the published reports. *JAMA* had unknowingly published one of those articles itself. In that article published in 2002, a Merck scientist was listed as the lead author, but nothing was disclosed about the ghostwritten contributors. Former *JAMA* editor Dr. Catherine DeAngelis said she felt "scammed." The editorial went on to say that Merck had "apparently manipulated dozens of publications to promote Vioxx," and that it was clear that "at least some of the authors played little direct role in the study or review, yet still allowed themselves to be named as authors."[14]

In 2010, another scandal erupted around the textbook *Recognition and Treatment of Psychiatric Disorders: A Psychopharmacology Handbook for Primary Care*. The book was published in 1999 and authored by two academic psychiatrists, Dr. Charles Nemeroff of the University of Miami and Dr. Alan F. Schatzbert, then chair of psychiatry at Stanford University. A Washington, D.C.–based watchdog group known as Project on Government Oversight (POGO) has informed the National Institutes of Health (NIH) about three publications, including the above textbook, in which GlaxoSmithKline (GSK) paid Scientific Therapeutics Information (STI), a marketing firm, to perform ghostwriting on drug benefits. "A draft of the textbook states it was sponsored by GSK and written by Diane M. Coniglio and Sally K. Laden of STI," POGO wrote. "In a letter addressed to Dr. Nemeroff, Ms. Laden provided an updated status of the textbook. Her timeline states that she wrote the first draft, which was then sent to Drs. Nemeroff and Schatzberg, the publisher, and GlaxoSmithKline. The timeline also notes that GSK was given all three drafts and was sent page proofs for final approval." The letter further stated, "We have discovered that the NIH gave $66.8 million in grants over the last five years to a handful of researchers who used ghostwriters for scientific publications." Drs. Nemeroff and Schatzberg had received $23.3 million in NIH grants over the past five years.[15] The documents revealing this information were uncovered in the discovery process of a lawsuit against GSK. In response, GSK and Drs. Nemeroff and Schatzberg, as well as the APA, have all claimed these are false allegations and that the book was peer-reviewed by multiple outside experts.[16]

CONTINUING MEDICAL EDUCATION (CME)

Doctors do not receive any training about drugs following medical school that is not funded, structured, and/or provided by the pharmaceutical industry. Every rep interaction, meeting, CME dinner program, lunch-n-learn, symposium, medical convention, and the like has been paid for and more than likely programmed by Pharma. This leaves little room for fair, balanced, third-party education concerning drugs once doctors are in practice.

Because the pharmaceutical industry's unilateral influence on continuing education raises concern about the objectivity and integrity of medical academic teaching, it would be valuable to review the history of medical education and how it has evolved hand-in-hand with pharmaceutical advertising in the 20th century. Health scholar Marc A. Rodwin of Suffolk University Law School has written a very useful historical account of the industry's influence on CME in his paper entitled "Drug Advertising, Continuing Medical Education, and Physician Prescribing Review: A Historical Review and Reform Proposal," in which he recommends a number of much-needed reforms.

The Accreditation Council for Continuing Medical Education (ACCME) was formed by the American Medical Association and six other organizations in 1980. The ACCME accredits companies that offer CME and authorizes other institutions and organizations to accredit CME providers. The ACCME also develops criteria to evaluate educational programs, which are used in accrediting CME providers. States requiring doctors to have CME generally specify that it must come from educational entities that they or the ACCME have accredited. Historically, there were only a few commercial firms that provided CME. However, these commercial CME providers also performed pharmaceutical marketing and public relations work. At the time ACCME was first formed, most CME was conducted by medical schools and societies.[17]

Commercially funded CME became a big hit among physicians wishing to defer the cost of their required continued education. By 2006, there were 158 for-profit CME providers largely resulting from pharmaceutical industry sponsorship. This was a rapid expansion from a meager 10 providers in 1980 and 68 in 2000. Accredited providers include medical schools, hospitals, health care systems, physician organizations, for-profit firms, nonprofit organizations, government entities, insurers, and other unclassified groups. In addition to accredited CME, pharmaceutical companies organize activities that are also deemed to be CME even when not accredited.[18]

Rodwin joins other critics of the 2004 ACCME guidelines, claiming they should be stricter. For example, the current guidelines state that a provider "cannot be required" by a sponsor to accept advice or direction regarding speakers, program content, or meaning. However, Rodwin maintains the current "language does not prohibit commercial supporters from offering advice, CME providers from soliciting suggestions from them, or CME providers voluntarily following suggestions of commercial supporters." He further states that his interviews with CME providers indicate that these occurrences are common practice.[19]

I can confirm many of Rodwin's assertions from my own personal experience working with CME programs. As a rep, I frequently organized hunting expeditions, fishing trips, golf outings, and other entertainment for my doctors and then coded and expensed the events, as instructed by management, as CME. Additionally, a product manager once instructed me to fire one of my doctors from the company's speaker's bureau after he had independently decided to utilize his own data and slides for a dinner CME presentation and contradicted my company's marketing message and product positioning. The manager was absolutely furious after the program, and he emphatically turned to me and said, "Did you hear what he just told your doctors? You'd better get into every one of those offices next week and do damage control, and *his* office better be your first call letting him know that if he doesn't want to play ball, there are plenty of folks who will!"

The United States isn't the only corner of the world where Pharma has gained ironclad control over medical education and journal reporting. In 2008, MSD—short for Merck, Sharp & Dohme—signed a partnership agreement with the British Medical Journal (BMJ) Group, effectively giving MSD control over 350 interactive learning courses in more than 20 medical therapy areas. Merck is the manufacturer of 13 different vaccines in addition to blockbuster pharmaceuticals such as the ill-fated Vioxx. Also worth noting is that it is the maker of the MMR vaccine, which has long been at the center of the autism controversy.[20]

Following that agreement in 2009, Univadis, a Merck trademark, entered into a CME partnership with yet another British medical journal, the *Lancet*, to provide medical education and an information website. It is easy to see here why there may be serious concern that Merck could potentially use its partnerships to discredit critics and squelch any controversy regarding risks uncovered with its products, as well as to unilaterally influence doctors' medical opinions and, ultimately, their prescribing habits by providing biased Merck education. The stated purpose of the Merck/BMJ/*Lancet* partnerships was to "change the face of medical education in Europe and beyond." The implications of that statement in terms of the safety and promotional campaign for mandatory drugs and vaccines for our children could be far and wide reaching in consequence!

PHARMA REPS: FRIEND OR FOE?

I enjoyed a long, successful career as a pharmaceutical rep. For the majority of the time, I was a specialty or hospital rep, so I received an extensive amount of advanced training that wasn't always available to the average field rep. If I learned anything in my tenure as a Pharma rep, it was that every relationship has a monetary value. I was taught how to distinguish with whom and where I would get the most bang for my buck early on. The rule of thumb was that 80 percent of sales came from 20 percent of the physician population. It was necessary not only to identify who constituted that 20 percent, but also to find ways to initially gain exposure to—and eventually the confidence of—that body of prescribers. I became an accomplished people profiler in order to win friends and better influence a doctor's prescribing habits.

Reps are initiated into the business with a sort of boot camp training in the corporate home offices. During that process, they are usually given several weeks of product information, sales training, corporate grooming, and psychological conditioning. That being said, Pharma reps emerge as masters of schmooze and relationship selling. The mantra of quid quo pro can be heard frequently in discussions among reps in waiting rooms and hallways. Or, as they say where I'm from, "You scratch my back, and I'll scratch yours!" More often than not, the obligation established between doctors and reps tends to be subtle and unspoken, but the bottom-line mentality exists for the sales rep all the same. I don't know one Pharma rep who could honestly say he or she hasn't bribed or outright strong-armed a doctor to influence his or her prescribing habits. I know I did it daily, and I wasn't some rogue rep who was following the beat of my own drummer. I was an accomplished, well-paid professional who learned fast and was considered to be exceptionally good at my job!

Unfortunately, my job was frequently masqueraded as education and was presumed to involve the presentation of fair, balanced information and research—especially in the institutional environments where doctors practice medicine and are trained by their superiors. However, there was a universal motivation common to all Pharma reps that belied that illusion. It was called sales quotas. And, I knew that the bottom line of what I was there to do was to increase sales of my company's product portfolio. I was given the money, tools, and means to do whatever it took to achieve those ends. Doctors were not necessarily the end users of my products, but they were the gatekeepers to those customers. I was trained very effectively on how to get through that gate with relationship-selling skills.

Toward the end of my career, because I was required to bring food in to so many of my appointments, I felt more like a food caterer than a sales rep! I eventually hired a caterer on retainer for emergencies so that I could call at the drop of a hat in order to have gourmet food delivered to my doctors' offices. Food, candy, promo items such as scratch pads and pens, trinkets, and gifts were the mainstay of my marketing armamentarium. I was a goodie girl, and I never went anywhere empty handed. I competed with other companies, not only on the merits of my drugs, but on the merits of my bribery methods as well. Because if all other promotional avenues failed, I had to figure out what I could do to effectively bribe the physician to prescribe my drugs without offending his/her sense of integrity, morality, or professional ethics.

As another former Pharma rep so aptly described the position, "It's [the pharmaceutical rep's] job to figure out what a physician's price is. For some, it's dinner at the finest restaurants; for others, it's enough convincing data to let them prescribe confidently; and for others, it's my attention and friendship . . . but at the most basic level, everything is for sale and everything is an exchange."[21] I couldn't have written a better job description for a Pharma rep myself.

PUBLIC SERVICE VERSUS PHARMA SERVICE ANNOUNCEMENTS

Raising public awareness generally translates to fear mongering and disease mongering for the pharmaceutical industry. If the ad references any type of treatment option available, it's an infomercial from Pharma and not a public service ad. Keep in mind, since the pharmaceutical industry is a capitalistic, for-profit industry, it isn't likely to pay out costly prime-time advertising dollars to inform you about anything that does not benefit them financially in doing so.

One can find multiple examples of public service campaigns initiated by the pharmaceutical industry to raise awareness about a specific disease state or mental disorder such as depression. The current marketing campaign for the use of antipsychotics in *treatment-resistant depression* is a perfect case in point. First, the manufacturers want to raise awareness in the public that many of the patients taking antidepressants aren't experiencing symptom relief. In other words, patients on antidepressants still have complaints of depressed mood, low energy, poor appetite, sleep disturbance, and so forth, despite the fact they are taking medication to treat the many symptoms that commonly accompany depression.* Next, the drug companies put out prime-time commercials on TV and place ads in popular magazines that let patients know that they are not alone in this dilemma: "In fact, 1 out of 3 people on antidepressants still suffer from depression." However, the good news is they now have another drug that you can add to your antidepressant treatment regimen, an atypical antipsychotic to be exact, and according to the ads, "MANY people experience improvement in as little as two weeks." Ask your doctor if Abilify/Seroquel/Risperdal/ Zyprexa is right for you!

My intelligence as a consumer is insulted by this advertising campaign; isn't yours? If the first drug isn't working, why don't they stop that treatment before they try anything else? I'll tell you why. It's because they don't want to acknowledge the serious complications that can be created in withdrawal from an antidepressant any more than they want to entertain the loss of income that recommendation would represent in the antidepressant market. Antipsychotics are designed to gain add-on business expansion in this marketing campaign, but they are not intended to replace the antidepressants . . . not just yet. This promotional campaign merely sets the stage for future events. According to the clinical meta-analyses, antidepressants don't work for the

---

* Patients who are proponents of antidepressants will swear by the drugs and how they helped improve their mood, which isn't surprising considering the substantial placebo effect seen with all of the antidepressant drug trials. It's the big, white elephant in the room that the pharmaceutical industry doesn't want to acknowledge. In the jargon of the industry, more and more antidepressant trials are *crossing the futility boundary*, meaning that even though some patients may have a positive response to the drug, nearly the same number of patients who took an inert placebo also reported a positive response.

majority of people, and most of the category blockbusters are quickly losing their patent protection. Manufacturers will be looking to transfer those markets to other patented products in the very near future.

PHARMA FRONT GROUPS: ASTROTURF OR GRASSROOTS?

In New Jersey, Bristol-Myers Squibb (BMS) funded the creation of a program called Mind Matters, designed "to reduce the stigma of mental illness." The Mind Matters program is being implemented throughout New Jersey in a number of Boys and Girls Clubs, and its stated purpose is to "empower children to seek help when needed." BMS is a global pharmaceutical manufacturer whose mission statement claims to "extend and enhance human life."[22] One has to question, however, whether or not Boys and Girls Clubs are the appropriate avenue for BMS to assist others in the identification of troubled youth who will then be referred to services and become psychiatric drug customers. Kids involved in these programs are known to be primarily from lower socioeconomic groups and children of color. They also tend to be members of single-parent families, resulting in inadequate adult supervision as well as Medicaid coverage. Translation: these children are potential cash cows for Pharma and will most likely be drugged.

National Alliance for the Mentally Ill

The National Alliance on Mental Illness (NAMI) was formed in 1979 and was originally called the National Alliance for the Mentally Ill. NAMI is a nationwide nonprofit organization that is well organized and well funded. They have affiliates in all 50 states in addition to the District of Columbia and Puerto Rico and can be found in thousands of local communities as well. NAMI's stated mission is to provide support, education, advocacy, and research for people and their families living with mental illness through various public education and awareness activities. However, NAMI also understands that its role as an educator serves a commercial end. In a document filed with the government by NAMI in 2000, it stated that "providers, health plans, and pharmaceutical companies want to grow their markets and to increase their share of the market . . . NAMI will cooperate with these entities to grow the market by making persons aware of the issues involving severe brain disorders."[23]

Just as the bipolar diagnostic expansion occurred when psychiatry split the old manic-depressive disorder into three separate bipolar categories, pharmaceutical companies and their advocates mounted massive educational campaigns to alert consumers. For example, Abbott Laboratories and NAMI teamed up to promote a "Bipolar Awareness Day."[24] Abbott is the manufacturer of the antiseizure drug, Depakote, which acquired Food and Drug Administration (FDA) approval for the treatment of acute bipolar mania in 1995. State organizations of NAMI published newsletters to educate members, professionals, and the public alike about bipolar illness and the potential of new drug treatments.

At the national level, NAMI provides strategic direction and resources to all of its affiliates. NAMI's advocacy and political muscle also extend to federal agencies and the White House.[25] Because of that, NAMI's activities and funding have come under scrutiny in recent years. In 2008, a prominent NAMI member accused the organization of a serious conflict of interest by not disclosing that they receive more than half of their funding from pharmaceutical manufacturers. In 2009, the *New York Times* reported that U.S. senator Grassley's investigation of this issue confirmed that more than 66 percent of NAMI's funding came from pharmaceutical manufacturers.[26] This is a grievous conflict of interest, considering that NAMI lobbies Congress and other federal agencies to obtain funding for expensive drug treatment protocols couching their interest as a grassroots advocacy group for the mentally ill rather than as a Pharma-sponsored mouthpiece for special interests—psychiatric drug interests!

Children and Adults with Attention Deficit Hyperactivity Disorder (CHADD)

Another interesting grassroots organization, called CHADD, has a strikingly similar advocacy model . . . and funding issue. CHADD purports itself to be a nonprofit advocacy, education, and support group for people affected by ADHD. In its 2008–2009 annual report, CHADD states that their continuing goal is to, "Disseminate and increase information about AD/HD to target audiences, which include parents and families, public policymakers, the media, African American leaders, Spanish language users, mental health and health care professionals, and educators."

CHADD's Conflict of Interest Policy specifically states that "a financial interest is not necessarily a conflict of interest." However, since its inception in 1988, Ciba-Geigy, the manufacturer of Ritalin, quietly contributed more than $1 million to underwrite CHADD in the form of grants and other valuable services. As reported in the Merrow Report aired on PBS on October 20, 1995, CHADD, was found to be distributing misleading information to hundreds of thousands of parents and professionals that exaggerated the benefits of drug therapy for ADHD—including Ciba-Geigy's drug, Ritalin.

For years, supported by Ciba-Geigy funding, CHADD lobbied the Drug Enforcement Administration (DEA) to reduce the classification of Ritalin from a Class II controlled substance to a Class III. That reclassification would have allowed Ciba-Geigy to produce more Ritalin without any government restrictions. Fortunately, following the airing of the Merrow Report, the DEA put a stop to those particular lobbying efforts. In 1996, Ciba-Geigy merged with Sandoz and formed Novartis Pharmaceuticals. My recent review of CHADD's website did not reveal any mention of Novartis or of the organization's financial conflict of interest or association with any of the other psychotropic drug manufacturers.

Direct-to-Consumer Advertising

Pharmaceutical manufacturers were delighted when new guidelines released by the FDA in 1997 loosened the rules for advertising directly to consumers. According to these guidelines, drug companies could fulfill their obligation to inform consumers about the risks of prescription pharmaceuticals in drug advertisements by referring to four additional sources of information: the patient's doctor, a toll-free number, a magazine or newspaper ad, and a website. TV ads then became a major source of marketing influence on consumers and the largest share of Pharma's advertising budget. The big question is, of course, whether drug advertising leads to improvements in public health or to the unnecessary spending and inappropriate diagnosis and treatment of so-called disease.

Despite claims by the pharmaceutical industry that direct-to-consumer advertising is beneficial, educational, and raises awareness, the public is actually often misled or deliberately misinformed by these ads according to Public Citizen, a health research group in Washington, D.C.[27] Direct-to-consumer advertising is a drug marketing anomaly known only in New Zealand and the United States. No other country in the world allows this practice. Slick Madison Avenue ads line the magazines consumers buy and peruse, prime-time radio and TV announcers tout medical advancements about which you need to "ask your doctor," and the media picks up Pharma press releases and prints their marketing spin as though it is the latest, greatest medical advancement to be scientifically proved. Yet, the average consumer is ill equipped to know the risk-to-benefit ratio of these products and is ill advised to be making these types of decisions based on advertising rather than fair, balanced information. Direct-to-consumer advertising promotes patient hypochondria and self-diagnosis. A late night bout of anxiety, after drinking coffee all day or consuming empty calories of carbohydrates and sugar all night, suddenly becomes restless leg syndrome in the TV viewer's mind. The end result is a special visit to their doctor and a request for a drug!

Overwhelmed parents and educators fall prey to these marketing tactics quite frequently. After all, has it not been proved that ADHD can be effectively treated with stimulants, thereby decreasing the disruption to the classroom and lives of others by these problematic, mentally ill kids? Has it been *established*? Yes, it most definitely has been established by both Pharma and the psychiatric industry that stimulants are an effective treatment for kids with ADHD. Consequently, millions of children are currently taking psychotropic drugs for ADHD symptom management. However, have stimulant drugs been *proved* to be an effective treatment in the long term? No. In fact, quite the opposite is true. Medication use was a marker for "greater increase in symptoms and decrease in overall function" in both years three and six of the highly touted, long-term, follow-up Multi-Modal Treatment for ADHD (MTA) study on stimulant use with ADHD kids.[28]

In addition to the disappointing long-term outcomes with ADHD stimulants, there have been numerous black-box warnings issued in recent years, and the exposure of fatal risks and fraudulent researchers and clinical trials that have overstated benefits with a number of psychiatric drugs being used in children. The risk-to-benefit equation clearly bodes against the use of these major pharmaceuticals to address the behavioral and psychological issues of our kids. Unfortunately, the numbers do not lie, and the real numbers tell a harrowing story of deception and harm perpetrated against parents and their children for the benefit of investment portfolios and corporate profits.

GOVERNMENT-MANDATED SCREENING/ TREATMENTS

Political Lobbying

I was constantly reminded by my product managers as a pharmaceutical rep that I needed to get more *voice share* in my territory. In other words, the competition in drug sales is really steep, and I was expected to be heard by the prescribing physician above and beyond the voices and activities of my competition in some way. In fact, that was the reasoning behind the hiring of so many part-time contract sales forces by the industry in the 1990s—to increase voice share.

However, the pharmaceutical industry knows that the most effective way for them to get more voice share in government is to man the corridors and legislative offices of the capital buildings throughout the nation with PhRMA (the Pharmaceutical Research and Manufacturers of America). Comprising one of the biggest lobbying staffs on K Street, PhRMA represents the interests of 32 brand-name drug manufacturers. They employ more than 3,000 lobbyists of which there are more than 300 in Washington, D.C., alone. More than a third of these lobbyists were former federal officials.[29] Political connections have helped drug companies to battle price constraints, stretch patent guidelines preventing generic infiltration, and protect manufacturers against litigation.

Pharmaceutical companies are worried about health care reform, and they are willing to pay big bucks to lobbyists in order to protect their interests. According to documents filed by PhRMA with the IRS, the drug industry's chief lobbyists raised and spent at least $101.2 million on advocacy efforts during the health care debate in 2009.[30] Apparently, "money talks" as the old saying goes. PhRMA was effective in blocking the import of drugs from Canada, which would be more cost effective to the American consumer, and in continuing to prevent any government price control or negotiation. The U.S. government, unlike many other countries, cannot negotiate better pricing for consumers by making bulk purchases from the pharmaceutical industry as it does with other businesses.

PhRMA's former CEO, Billy Tauzin, was quoted as saying that year, "We're working with groups we never worked with before—Families USA, the American Agenda, labor, health care providers—that never stood together on the same platform. We have every business reason to want to see this happen, and we have every moral reason to see this happen, because our patients are our first concern." I probably wouldn't be so skeptical about the truth of the intentions behind this man's statements and efforts if I didn't know that he was also the former Louisiana state congressman, who, before giving up his government post that gave PhRMA blanket control over Medicare drug pricing, influenced the current legislation. I dare say that price-gouged taxpayers and the Medicare program substantiates the claim that "patients [are the pharmaceutical manufacturers'] first concern."[31]

According to a study done by Boston University professors Alan Sager and Deborah Socolar in 2003, a total of 61 percent of Medicare money spent on prescription drugs will become profit for drug companies. The study predicted that pharmaceutical manufacturers would receive $139 billion in increased profits over an eight-year period. The Medicare prescription drug benefit started in 2006. The U.S. government contributes more money to the development of new drugs—in the form of tax breaks and subsidies—than any other government in the world. Nine of the 20 largest pharmaceutical corporations are based in the United States, yet drugs are more expensive here than anywhere else in the world. U.S. manufacturers produce 60 to 70 percent of the world's new pharmaceuticals.[32]

In 2011, the pharmaceutical industry gained a powerful new ally and voice to add to their choir in government. And it was an unlikely voice at that—former, nine-term congressman Bart Stupak. Stupak, once chairman of the House Energy and Commerce Committee's Oversight and Investigation Subcommittee, was known for his watchdog approach to the pharmaceutical industry, including probes into the FDA's handling of Baxter's drug Heparin that harmed hundreds and killed several people; investigating Merck and Schering-Plough for the late release of their data showing unfavorable outcomes for their cholesterol drug, Vytorin; and reprimanding Pfizer for producing misleading TV ads for its cholesterol-lowering drug, Lipitor. Stupak has now signed on as a legislative and government affairs partner with Venable, a law firm that has a sizable practice serving drug and medical device manufacturers. In a statement released to the press, Stupak was quoted as saying, "I'm excited about helping my new colleagues and the firm's clients to navigate choppy congressional waters."[33]

Pharma's lobbying efforts to influence government policy do not stop at drug pricing or drug availability. The pharmaceutical manufacturers want to utilize government policy and its authority to force unsuspecting members of the population to consume their products regardless of whether they want to and regardless of whether it is beneficial to them. The acquisition of key allies within government circles can prove invaluable to Pharma in its ability to influence policy, promote mandatory market expansion, and fund new drug approvals. This arm of the marketing plan is particularly important since drug manufacturers have identified their most lucrative expansion drug markets to be in mandated treatment, such as vaccines and psychiatric drugs, and their most lucrative expansion demographic, unfortunately, to be our children.

TEEN SCREEN: TEST OR TRAP?

To screen or not to screen? That is the question haunting many dubious parents and educators regarding the Teen Screen initiatives surfacing in schools and campuses around the nation. Teen Screen is another "Astroturf organization that has raised the eyebrows (and dander) of mental health activists and child advocates alike. The program's premise is to screen American kids for their potential risk for suicide and to facilitate the diagnosis and treatment of mental disorders via a short questionnaire. A close examination of the origin of Teen Screen and its sponsors suggests that the objective of Teen Screen is more than just a screening tool used to identify children at risk. It is clearly a Pharma-backed marketing ploy designed to increase the market share and use of psychotropic drugs in teens and children. In the same way I once plied busy medical staff members and doctors with food and trinkets as a pharmaceutical rep, Teen Screen lures youngsters as young as nine years old to test as potential customers for their wares by handing out movie tickets, food coupons, and pizza parties to eager participants. And it is done right in the child's school, often without parental consent.

Never mind that the vast majority of Teen Screen tests produce false positives for mental illness. The percentage of false positives for the Columbia Suicide Screen (CSS) is 84 percent, whereas the Diagnostic Predictive Scales (DPS) computer screen produces up to 94 percent false positives for mental illness.[34] Never mind that the stigma of one of these false diagnoses might haunt a child for the rest of his or her life. For example, children who have taken stimulant drugs past the age of 12 are not permitted into the U.S. armed forces. Never mind that there are no scientific tests to validate or invalidate any diagnoses made based on the exam. Never mind that *the child's mind* may pay the ultimate price for having been the recipient of a psychotropic drug regimen during a critical developmental phase, even though it was entirely unwarranted.

Even in the recent wake of several black-box warnings required by the FDA and the tremendous body of data revealing the inefficacy and dangers of psychotropic drugs used in children, the pharmaceutical industry continues their covert marketing campaigns with front organizations such as Teen Screen. This serves to delude the public into thinking that these treatments are both safe and effective to use in teen suicide prevention and that they should continue to be forced on our kids, when, in fact, many of the reported suicides and homicides involving either teens or adolescents are alleged to be the direct result of adverse effects of a psychotropic drug and have been attributed to drug use, rather than the lack thereof. In 2009, the NIH and the FDA released a study that found that children and teens that died suddenly were 7.4 times more likely to have been on stimulant medications.[35]

Teen Screen was established in Tulsa, Oklahoma, in 1997. As reported in a 2003 *Tulsa World* newspaper article, the executive director of the Mental Health Association in Tulsa was quoted as saying, "To the best of my knowledge, this is the highest number of youth suicides we've ever had during the school year—a number we find very frightening." This, to put it mildly, leaves one to question the effectiveness of Teen Screen.

MARKET EXPANSION TECHNIQUES: OFF-LABEL MARKETING PRACTICES FOR PSYCHOTROPICS

The off-label marketing of drugs—or the promotion of drugs for indications not approved by the FDA—is a common, albeit illegal marketing tactic. Off-label marketing tactics are often employed after a manufacturer discovers through a competitor's clinical trials or the public's general use that a drug has beneficial side effects that can be utilized for the treatment of other health problems. For example, the atypical antipsychotics are known to be highly sedating; therefore, doctors will prescribe them as a sleep aid. This is an off-label indication since the FDA has not granted its approval for that use. However, it is important to distinguish that doctors can legally prescribe drugs for whatever indications they deem appropriate. It is only illegal for the manufacturers to *promote* drugs off-label.

The FDA approved Abilify for use in adolescent patients with schizophrenia or bipolar mania in 2007. This was the precedent that unleashed an avalanche of competitive off-label marketing of antipsychotic drugs to children. Drug companies will often claim that a *class effect* exists in regard to a benefit, especially if one of their competitors receives an expanded label approval and larger target market. This happened when Abilify received an adolescent bipolar indication. By definition, a class effect is when all the drugs in a particular class have the same activity or benefit. In other words, the assumption is that if one drug has a specific benefit, then all the drugs belonging to that same pharmacological class should also have that benefit. Since Abilify received its pediatric label expansion, similar approval has been given for Seroquel, Risperdal, and Zyprexa, thereby granting the legal promotion for the use of antipsychotics in kids by nearly all of the manufacturers. Only Geodon has yet to receive approval for the treatment of youth disorders. As a result, atypical antipsychotics have become the number one drug category and income earner in pharmaceutical sales two consecutive years running. In both 2008 and 2009, antipsychotic manufacturers sold $14.6 billion each year.[36]

Now there is controversy about whether Abilify is even effective for the maintenance treatment of bipolar illness at all. *PLoS Medicine* published a paper in early May 2011 that challenged the original 2003 Abilify study that had garnered Abilify's label expansion for the maintenance treatment of bipolar disorder. First released in the *American Journal of Psychiatry,* the study came under closer scrutiny by researchers due to a number of shortcomings. First, the authors state that the duration of the trial was too short to establish that Abilify maintained the initial benefit or assisted in preventing mood swings long term.

Secondly, there was a high discontinuation rate with very few patients actually completing the trial. Third, the trial was based on a small group of patients who demonstrated an initial response to Abilify, making it difficult to extrapolate findings to a larger group of patients with bipolar disorder. Lastly, the trial design took patients abruptly off of Abilify, which had been administered to them during a previous run-in phase, and then reassigned them to the placebo arm. So, any differences seen between risks for relapse between the trial arms may also reflect the harmful effects seen with *rapid drug withdrawal* in patients assigned to placebo.

According to one of the *PLoS* authors, Nicholas Rosenlicht, this deeply flawed trial has been cited with virtually no criticism as evidence supporting the use of Abilify for this indication despite the fact that Abilify does not demonstrate a long-term benefit over placebo. And, as Rosenlicht concludes, "it appears that marketing information, rather than science, has driven the rapid adoption of Abilify as an accepted agent for the long-term treatment of bipolar disorder."[37] Consequently, it also appears that the manufacturers who marketed their antipsychotic drugs off label for the maintenance of patients with bipolar disorder, substantiating that use based on an assumed class effect, in reality had very flimsy scientific evidence to support doing so. Therefore, the risk-to-benefit ratio for bipolar patients treated with antipsychotics has significantly increased.

The past several years have been tough for the pharmaceutical industry in terms of the compensatory legal action taken by states and individuals against them for their illegal, off-label marketing practices. Many of these lawsuits were the result of Pharma's illegal marketing of psychotropic drugs for children. For example, Forest Laboratories pleaded guilty and paid more than $313 million in 2009 to settle a Department of Justice investigation for its off-label promotion of Celexa and Lexapro for kids—even though the FDA had rejected these drugs for use in children and, additionally, European data had shown that neither drug was useful in children or youths. However, lawsuits alleged that pharmaceutical sales reps recommended crushing up the tablets into apple sauce in order to make them more palatable for children.[38] This is a tactic I was also trained to use in overcoming a pediatrician's objections to the administration of foul-tasting antibiotics children didn't want to take.

The lawsuits further alleged that Forest overcame resistance to the pediatric use of its antidepressants by bribing doctors. Among the goodies of cash and gifts that Forest reportedly handed out, many via their sales force, were the following:

- Tickets to St. Louis Cardinals games
- A $1,000 certificate to Alain Ducasse, an exclusive, expensive restaurant in New York
- A trip to see a George Carlin concert
- $1,000 in cash to attend dinner at the Doral Park Country Club in Miami
- A trip to the Great Escape amusement park in New York
- Tickets to *The Nutcracker* at a playhouse in New Jersey[39]

This example involved the marketing of antidepressants to pediatricians. However, there have been a multitude of lawsuits in recent years filed against major pharmaceutical manufacturers for the off-label promotion of their antipsychotic drugs to children.

In October 2010, the *New York Times* published an in-depth article entitled "Side Effects May Include Lawsuits," which cataloged a number of recent lawsuits. In 2007, BMS paid $515 million to settle state and federal investigations into the marketing of its antipsychotic Abilify to child psychiatrists and nursing homes. However, BMS did not admit to any wrongdoing. According to a government filing in 2010, Pfizer also paid more than 250 child psychiatrists to promote its antipsychotic Geodon even though the drug was only approved in adults.[40] Eli Lilly was investigated not only for off-label marketing activity in nursing homes but also for training its reps to rebut valid medical concerns about its antipsychotic Zyprexa. According to the Justice Department, Lilly produced a video called "The Myth of Diabetes" and had its reps use it to sell Zyprexa. Zyprexa became a blockbuster drug despite its problematic side effect profile of inducing premature death in the elderly and of producing serious metabolic issues—including diabetes![41] In 2010, AstraZeneca became the fourth major drug company in three years to settle a government investigation with a whopping fine for what has been described by federal officials as an array of illegal promotions of antipsychotics for children, the elderly, veterans, and prisoners. Still, the payment of $520 million that AstraZeneca was required to make only amounted to 2.4 percent of the $21.6 billion made on Seroquel sales from 1997 to 2009.[42] In other words, these fines equated to the mere cost of doing business!

CLINICAL STANDARDS OF CARE: PLAYING THE NUMBERS

Clinical standards of care are the protocols by which doctors are insured and medicine is commonly practiced. Medical conditions are defined by a set of numbers, and if the range of those numbers increases even slightly, then all of a sudden millions of patients can become candidates for treatment overnight—simply by adjusting the scale and the resulting medical protocol.

A perfect case in point would be the cholesterol story about certain number ranges for LDL and HDL and their associated risk for heart attack. When I sold Pravachol (pravastatin) for BMS, I was required to know the statin clinical studies inside and out. Interestingly enough, after Lipitor was launched and became my product's biggest competitor, the other statin manufacturers (BMS included) began to lobby to have the clinical guidelines for treatment adjusted. New data suggested that lowering LDL more than 130 mg/dl would improve cardiovascular outcomes. As a result, the new guidelines swiftly became the new clinical standard, and the population of patients eligible for statin treatment increased from 12 million to more than 36 million–over night!

Now the pharmaceutical industry is expanding its statin market to include our children. Remember, these drugs are not tried on children in their clinical phases, so there is no short-or long-term data available on their efficacy or safety in children. Yet, statin drugs are now recommended prophylactically for children as young as eight years of age. We will only know the ramifications of this down the road, as cholesterol is the most common organic molecule in the entire body and brain and is needed for every biochemical process that we have, especially in the developing bodies and minds of our children.

EVERGREENING AND THE TRANSFER OF PATIENTS TO PATENT-PROTECTED PRODUCTS

Finally, once a pharmaceutical has become a blockbuster drug and then loses its patent, generic competition begins to seriously erode the branded drug's profit margin. It is then time for the manufacturer to transfer the patient population to a newer, branded product. Many examples of this exist in the psychiatric drug market. One such example is the launch of Sarafem for the newly invented premenstrual mood dysphoric disorder just as Prozac was about to go off patent. Sarafem contains the exact same chemical entity as Prozac but is packaged in a purple and pink capsule.

I personally participated in this same marketing tactic with the introduction of Haldol Decanoate in the 1980s. A full-court press marketing campaign was unleashed with the product launch in an attempt to transfer business from the Haldol tablet form to the branded, much more expensive Haldol Decanoate delivery form. Despite the increased side effect profile and exorbitant difference in cost to both the consumer and public assistance programs such as Medicaid and the Veterans Administration, Haldol Decanoate quickly absorbed large portions of the market that were previously held by the tablet form. The average wholesale cost of a Haldol Decanoate injection at that time was $165 per injection, whereas Haldol tablets sold for mere pennies on the dollar.

The SSRI antidepressants first came under congressional scrutiny in 1991. Since that time, there have been two additional hearings prompting the addition of black-box warnings and warning expansions to be issued for the prescribers and consumers of these drugs. In addition, many of the previous blockbusters such as Prozac, Zoloft and Paxil have lost, or are about to lose, their exclusive patent rights and are subject to infiltration by generic competition. Meanwhile, a very large percentage of patients have complained that they do not receive any benefit from their antidepressant drugs and remain depressed even after months of treatment. Enter the *treatment-resistant depression* expansion market. This ingenious marketing tactic actually blames the patient for the inefficacy of the patient's antidepressant drug! It's a savvy, add-on business technique, as one drug conveniently creates a problem for which another drug can then be prescribed in addition to the antidepressant, but it cannot be used as a stand-alone treatment. This prevents the patient from discontinuing the first drug that isn't working and replacing it with something else. The new treatment is simply added on.

MILKING THE CASH COWS

Chemical Restraints for Incarcerated Kids/Residential Treatment Facilities/Foster Kids/Medicaid Rosters

It is also startling to witness the increase in the number of children labeled as learning disabled or diagnosed with *disruptive behavior disorders* in recent years. These children generally receive their schooling in special education programs. Federal spending for special education grew from $1 billion in 1977 to $30 billion by 1994. The 1991 expansion of the Individuals with Disabilities Education Act to include ADD as "another health impaired" category was a huge contributor to this increase.[43]

Money that was appropriated by Congress primarily to aid indigent children with severe physical disabilities, such as cerebral palsy, Down syndrome, deafness, blindness, and so on, now largely finances children with common learning and behavioral disabilities such as ADHD and delayed speech. Inadvertently, it has also created a financial motive for many needy parents to seek prescriptions for powerful psychotropic drugs who may not otherwise have requested them for their children (case in point, the overdose death in 2006 of little Rebecca Riley, a four-year-old child who had been treated for bipolar disorder since the age of two).

A three-part series published in the *Boston Globe* in 2010 alleged the existence of troubling incentives that could pose risk to children. This launched a congressional investigation into whether too many children were being given psychotropic drugs as a means of proving the severity level of their disability, which would qualify them to receive up to $700 a month plus Medicaid benefits. Statistics show that out of the 1.2 million low-income children who receive SSI benefits, 53 percent, or 640,000, qualify because of mental disabilities—up from 8 percent in 1990. By significant margins, delayed speech and ADHD were the majority reasons children received benefits.[44]

Educational institutions are eligible to receive funding for every learning disabled child in the school system. In some states, such as my home state of Texas, schools are permitted to throw out the test scores of learning disabled children. This improves the numbers when calculating the institution's academic performance scores for purposes of funding, certification, and other credentials. Today, it is not unusual for a school district to have one out of every four of its students in special education one way or another.[45]

I worked in the Texas foster care system for five years as a volunteer court-appointed special advocate for abused and neglected children who had been thrust into the foster care system. It was during this time that I identified more than one financial incentive for labeling and drugging our children. Foster parents often *pushed* me to advocate for their wards to be drugged, not only in an attempt to control the children's behavior but also as an avenue for increased monetary compensation. Children diagnosed with mental illness and placed on medication while they are in state care reap a higher level of reimbursement for their foster families, residential facilities, or other caretakers.

It was my observation that very young children—some as young as two and three years old—were routinely placed on psychiatric medications almost immediately after entering the system. Most frequently, the kids were given these powerful chemicals for off-label indications. This alarmed me because as a rep who had sold an older antipsychotic that competed with many of the drugs I saw in children's charts, I knew that most of these drugs had never been clinically tried and/or approved in children. Even more remarkable to me as a taxpayer was that these kids covered by Medicaid were being prescribed the most expensive, newer, branded drugs available on the psychiatric market.

This led me to further investigate the now burning question in my mind, Why?

In the release of a groundbreaking yearlong investigation conducted by Youth Today, ample evidence was documented that American youth are receiving potent, atypical antipsychotic drugs that are indicated for schizophrenia and bipolar illness when most of these kids have not been given either diagnosis. Therefore, these drugs are being prescribed for off-label conditions for which the drugs have not been tested and/or proved effective. The Youth Today findings were derived from records submitted by state juvenile systems nationwide that documented the use of atypical antipsychotics for a wide variety of indications, including intermittent explosive disorder, oppositional defiant disorder, and ADHD, among others.[46]

From 1996 to 2006, prescriptions for psychiatric drugs increased more than 50 percent among children. During that same time frame, mental health care spending increased by 30 percent due, by a large degree, to psychiatric drug expenditures.[47] In fact, the U.S. Department of Health and Human Services reported that in 2006 more money was spent on the treatment of mental disorders for children ages 0 to 17 than on any other medical condition—a total of $8.9 billion. It is estimated that 69 cents out of each dollar spent on antipsychotic medications in the United States comes out of the taxpayer's pocket. New federally financed drug research reveals a stark disparity: children in the public system are given powerful antipsychotic medicines at a rate four times higher than children whose parents have private insurance. Moreover, children covered by Medicaid are more likely to readily receive these drugs for less severe conditions than their middle-class counterparts.[48]

But the most disturbing data comes from a 16-state study from Rutgers University on the use of antipsychotics in children and adolescents covered by Medicaid, which reported that foster children received antipsychotic medications at a rate almost nine times that of other children covered by Medicaid.[49]

When you follow the money trail, it soon becomes clear that the pharmaceutical industry has mastered the art of lobbying the U.S. legislature. As the purse strings on the economy tighten, and fewer Americans have health insurance and can afford exorbitant drug prices, Pharma increases its activity in government and markets to our legislators in the form of lobbying. This bypasses the consumer completely and secures taxpayer funding to purchase mandated treatments that can then be imposed on the population in the name of good public health policies. These are marketing dollars well spent and produce a win-win situation for Pharma since the government does not negotiate pricing with the pharmaceutical industry for the end consumer and is content to pay whatever price the industry deems appropriate. Furthermore, this ensures that a steady increase in the purchase of certain products can be anticipated, regardless of economic variables, thereby stabilizing an otherwise volatile market for corporate investors.

CONCLUSION

This complex corporate initiative to create a lucrative, untapped expansion market for antipsychotic drugs was well planned, intentionally orchestrated, and skillfully executed. But for those of you who may prefer to have it spelled out concisely, here it is in a nutshell.

The pharmaceutical industry discovered that a couple of its psychiatric drug categories had a particularly high incidence of inducing a serious side effect known as *mania*. The SSRI and SNRI antidepressants, as well as ADHD stimulant drugs, can often create symptoms that are then unwittingly diagnosed by practitioners as bipolar disorder. Although, historically, bipolar illness was known only in adult populations, key opinion leaders and academic researchers established the PBD diagnosis as commonplace. This created an expansion market for the newer, branded atypical antipsychotics that were much more expensive than many of the older competing drugs already available generically. These influential individuals substantiated the validity of PBD by publishing articles and research in prestigious peer-reviewed journals, and antipsychotic manufacturers promoted their work via outlets of CME and other stealth marketing campaigns. Reps helped to further establish the routine use of the drugs with continual reiteration of the problem and by painting the perfect patient picture for physicians via their sales presentations—as well as with literal bribery—and encouraged the off-label use of antipsychotics for children.

Public service announcements were used to raise public awareness about the existence of the previously unrecognized PBD problem. Then, direct-to-consumer advertising was used to securely establish the problem in the minds of the consumer with television, radio, magazine, and newspaper ads. Pharma front organizations, such as NAMI, cleverly disguised as grassroots patient advocates, also decried the growing problem and need for increased availability of these questionable treatments for our kids—despite the serious risks involved and the absence of any long-term clinical efficacy data.

Lobbyists and congressmen proposed legislation that would mandate the screening of school children and infants for potential mental illness and helped not only to identify and label Pharma's customers, but also to ensure that those patients would receive the most expensive, branded treatments available through programs established for children treated while in state custody or in state supervision programs such as the Texas Medication Algorithm Project (TMAP). TMAP guaranteed the pharmaceutical industry that the prices of their newer antipsychotics would not be subjected to negotiation like pricing is with private contractors such as hospitals and HMOs. The cost is absorbed almost in its entirety by either private insurance or public tax dollars.

The FDA and other government agencies have been complicit in the problem, first, by approving pediatric and adolescent indications with the atypical antipsychotics using clinical efficacy data obtained from a few questionable manufacturer-sponsored trials, and second, by not clearly identifying and warning both prescribers and consumers about the causal relationship between previous psychotropic drug use and the emergence of the so-called bipolar epidemic among children. The final outcome of this highly sophisticated marketing campaign has been the profit-driven drugging of our country's most precious and most valuable resource—our children!

PART II
Drugging Our Children: Ethical and Legal Considerations

5

Pediatric Antipsychotics: A Call for Ethical Care

Jacqueline A. Sparks and Barry L. Duncan

Having heard all of this, you may choose to look the other way . . . but you can never say again that you did not know.
—William Wilberforce, Address to the English
Parliament Regarding the Slave Trade

A mother has a moment of panic, spying her daughter's arms criss-crossed with red cuts. Heartsick, she recalls a recent *Newsweek* article about bipolar illness and children. Could her child's boundless energy be mania and now this, depression? Where to turn? She picks up a phone book, scanning the yellow pages under *p* for *psychologist.*

A harried teacher does a double take when the behavior of a typi-cally disruptive middle schooler takes a bizarre turn. One minute he has his head on his desk, and the next, she spies him out the window shimmied halfway up the flagpole. All she can think as she rushes to the office is "this kid needs help!"

Young parents are at a loss to explain the uncontrollable rages of their five year old. As the mother barricades herself in the bedroom until his tantrum wears out, she remembers a family story of her great-uncle not being right. The preschool teacher's report about behavior problems suddenly takes on new meaning.

In each case, the specter of mental illness hovers. In each case, the fam-ily, a mental health professional, and others—teachers, social work-ers, and helpers—are drawn together in a reactive network. Decisions need to be made and a path charted, and time is critical. The decision faced by the clinician at this point represents a unique ethical dilemma. How the first professionals respond—what assessments are conducted, treatment plans developed, and recommendations made—has immediate and far-reaching consequences. The aftermath of these early decisions means no less than how the child comes to view his or her identity and whether relationships, school, and eventual career and civic work will be domains of competence or failure. They may mean the difference between a lifetime of health or chronic disability.

In the scenarios described, the likelihood that the child will be diagnosed with a mental disorder leading to a prescription of an antipsychotic is high. Would this possibility harm or help? Is this solution the best of available options? Is it ethical? Client welfare is the core of ethical practice in all mental health professions. Embedded in this is the centuries-old Hippocratic maxim to first do no harm. Additionally, all mental health practitioners are bound to give the best available information to clients to help them decide among various treatment options. Do no harm and informed consent form the centerpieces of ethical mental health practice. We believe that psychologists and other mental health practitioners hold these principles inviolable and work diligently to adhere to them. Our question, and one addressed in this chapter, is whether efforts to act ethically in challenging circumstances such as those described above achieve their intended purpose. What guidelines do clinicians have to chart a course that does the least harm and maximizes the chance that the young person can live a full and rewarding life? Finally, who decides what passes for do no harm and informed consent?

SCIENCE AND ETHICS

Antipsychotics are increasingly prescribed for teenagers, school-age children, and even preschoolers[1] to treat a growing array of problems including irritability, tantrums, aggression, mood dysregulation, and hyperactivity, in spite of the fact that there is no compelling research to support their use for these indications.[2] In many instances antipsychotics are being prescribed off label and for symptoms and diagnoses that don't involve psychosis. Moreover, multidrug cocktails consisting of various combinations of stimulants, antidepressants, and anticonvulsants in addition to antipsychotics are common.[3] Children often leave psychiatrists' or primary physicians' offices with a prescription that was not based on a mental health assessment and without a referral for psychotherapy.[4] Help, more and more, means a psychiatric drug and, all too often, several in combination.

Disturbingly, there is evidence that poor children are more likely to receive an antipsychotic prescription than their more fortunate counterparts.[5] According to a recent study, children covered by Medicaid are prescribed antipsychotics at a rate four times higher than those with private insurance and for less serious conditions.[6] In addition, there is disconcerting evidence about the extent of antipsychotic use with youth incarcerated in American juvenile detention centers. A groundbreaking, yearlong investigation published by *Youth Today* found that many incarcerated youths are getting these potent drugs, even without a diagnosis of schizophrenia or bipolar disorder.[7] Most often, the drugs are prescribed for diagnoses of intermittent explosive, oppositional defiant, and attention-deficit/hyperactivity disorders. According to the survey, more than a quarter of the prescriptions were written for youths who had no diagnosis. In other words, antipsychotics appear to serve as behavior management tools in these facilities— chemical restraints substituting for now banned physical restraints. Given that only 16 states responded to the *Youth Today* survey, including many with the largest state-held juvenile populations, the real extent of this practice is unknown.

How have antipsychotics become a first-line option for so many vulnerable children and adolescents, especially since these drugs have long been reserved for adult psychoses? Many clinicians and the public— parents, caregivers, teachers, and others grappling with how to address troubling child and adolescent behaviors—would likely say that the drugs are safe and effective and that scientific studies prove this. The scientist-practitioner and practitioner-scholar models and evidence-based practice require that intervention be supported by sound empirical research, ensuring that treatments are not likely to cause harm and are expected to help.[8] Presumably, when clinicians follow evidence-based guidelines, ethics is not a concern. Based on this common wisdom, burgeoning pediatric antipsychotic prescription is scientifically grounded and therefore ethical.

Let's examine this assumption—that science provides a solid foundation for the practice of pediatric psychotropic prescription. How well does the science hold up under scrutiny? Put another way, does current science provide an empirically and ethically valid case for placing so many children on powerful drugs? Several years ago, the American Psychological Association (APA) Working Group on Psychoactive Medications for Children and Adolescents looked at this very question.[9] Specifically, they examined whether the benefits of antipsychotics outweigh the risks for the under-18 age group. After a comprehensive investigation of the scientific literature, they found that studies supporting the use of antipsychotics to treat children were plagued with methodological limitations, including small sample sizes, open trials, and lower tier evidence (e.g., retrospective chart reviews and case reports). Moreover, they found an alarming picture of side effects. Many children participating in antipsychotic trials experienced some combination of somnolence, involuntary movement, cognitive impairment, elevated prolactin, intracardiac conduction, neuroleptic malignant syndrome, polycystic ovarian syndrome, weight gain, and general metabolic disorders, including type 2 diabetes mellitus, and transaminase elevation.[10]

Young people appear particularly susceptible to weight gain and associated cardiometabolic effects. One study found that 257 children and adolescents aged 4–19 added 8 to 15 percent of their weight in less than 12 weeks on either aripiprazole (Abilify), olanzapine (Zyprexa), quetiapine (Seroquel), or risperidone (Risperdal).[11] Wayne Goodman, head of a Food and Drug Administration (FDA) advisory panel on the pediatric antipsychotics, described the degree of weight gain in this trial as "alarming . . . the magnitude is stunning."[12] In an editorial accompanying the study,[13] Christopher Varley (Seattle Children's Hospital) and Jon McClellan (University of Washington School of Medicine) wrote that weight gain and changes in blood fat levels early in life have "ominous long-term health implications".

These data confirm prior findings that children and adolescents are highly vulnerable to antipsychotic medication–induced weight gain and metabolic adverse effects. The magnitude of weight gain is particularly concerning, as is the implication that metabolic adverse events may be underestimated in studies in which participants have had prior atypical antipsychotic medication exposure. Furthermore, the development of clinically significant hyperlipidemias and insulin resistance after only 12 weeks of treatment portends severe long-term metabolic and cardiovascular sequelae.

They concluded that the results of the study "challenge the widespread use of atypical antipsychotic medications in youth".

Adding to this grim picture, second-generation (atypical) antipsychotics do not appear to have a clear advantage over older ones when it comes to movement disorders, despite popular belief. In a recent, well-designed study with adults diagnosed with mood disorders or schizophrenia, rates of tardive dyskinesia (abnormal movements) for those taking second-generation antipsychotics (but naïve to conventional antipsychotics) were similar to those taking the older drugs.[14] Moreover, the incidence and prevalence of tardive dyskinesia in clinical practice, despite the widespread use of the newer drugs, remains unchanged from the 1980s. "It's definitely sad news for the patients," Scott Woods, lead author from Yale University Department of Psychiatry commented.[15] Movement disorders consistently surface in clinical trials of pediatric antipsychotics and at rates significantly greater than placebo, though they are rarely highlighted in article discussion sections or subsequent press releases.[16] No one has studied the long-term impact of these drugs on a developing nervous system. But even in the short term, one can only imagine how a stigmatizing and debilitating movement condition might sabotage a youth trying to succeed in school and at home.

‘ Two recent reports of the National Institute of Mental Health (NIMH)–funded Treatment of Early Onset Schizophrenia Spectrum Disorders study (TEOSS)[17] provide more evidence of an unfavorable risk/benefit profile for pediatric antipsychotic use. This trial compared the efficacy, tolerability, and safety of two second-generation antipsychotics (risperidone, or Risperdal, and olanzapine, or Zyprexa) to a first-generation antipsychotic (molindone, or Moban) for youths, ages 8–19, diagnosed with early onset schizophrenia spectrum disorder. At the end of 8 weeks, the liberally defined response rate was 50 percent for those treated with Moban, 46 percent for Risperdal, and 34 percent for Zyprexa.[18] Participants in the study were allowed concomitant use of antidepressants, anticonvulsants, and benzodiazepines, making it difficult to determine what actually accounted for even these disappointing findings. During the trial, a 17-year-old boy committed suicide, and an unspecified number of participants were hospitalized due to suicidality or worsening psychosis. These events are particularly disturbing in light of the fact that youths considered at risk for suicide were excluded from the study. Weight gain was deemed serious enough to warrant suspension of the Zyprexa arm. Adverse events were frequent in all three groups.

Youths who responded during the initial 8 weeks—47 of the 116— were entered into the 44-week maintenance study.[19] Seven other youths who did not meet responder criteria but had "sufficiently improved" according to the investigators, were allowed to continue, making a total of 54 participants in this phase of the trial. Forty of these dropped out during this period because of "adverse effects" or "inadequate response." Thus, only 14 of the 116 youths (12%) who entered the study responded to the medication and stayed on it for as long as one year. The optimistic wish that this well-heeled study would allay the fears of many, especially in light of rising rates of prescriptions, was dashed. Instead, TEOSS findings have fueled mounting concerns that the cost relative to benefit of these drugs for youth is too high.

It is hard, in fact, to locate any pediatric antipsychotic research to bolster a pro-antipsychotic case. An oft-cited series of studies examining the safety and efficacy of Risperdal for children diagnosed with autism reveals a familiar pattern of flaws that raise serious questions regarding author claims of efficacy and safety.[20] For example, the Risperdal trials (as well as all pediatric antipsychotic studies) did not use active placebos (sugar pills that mimic the side effects of active drugs). Without a placebo that feels like the real thing, youth, caretakers, and clinical raters likely can tell who is taking the actual drug and who isn't, effectively compromising the double blind and giving an unfair advantage to the drug. This is particularly problematic for the Risperdal trials as many trial participants recruited were not naïve to antipsychotic treatment. In other words, they knew well how it felt to be on the drugs and could readily determine if they were on them or not. Second, followup studies employed an abrupt drug withdrawal design to create the placebo group. This meant that children who were stable on the drug were shifted abruptly to placebo. Withdrawal symptoms experienced by children taken quickly off the active drug were labeled relapse and proof that the antipsychotic was needed for the longer term. Sedated children generally are not acting out or bothersome and score lower on scales that rate these types of behaviors. When we look at patient-rated measures, a different story emerges. For example, in the 2008 study of aripiprazole (Abilify) for youth aged 13–17 diagnosed with schizophrenia,[21] no differences were found between placebo and both drug groups (10 mg and 30 mg aripiprazole) on the total score of the *patient-rated* measure (Pediatric Quality of Life Enjoyment and Satisfaction Questionnaire). In other words, the measure that assessed how the teenagers felt they were doing in their lives, *from their perspectives,* failed to distinguish drug from placebo conditions.[22]

Finally, the duration of many pediatric antipsychotic studies is hardly adequate to determine the impact of these drugs on children over time. Aripiprazole (Abilify) was approved by the FDA for children between the ages of 10 and 17 for mania associated with bipolar I on the basis of one four-week trial. Approval for use of risperidone (Risperdal) for adolescents experiencing psychotic-type symptoms was based on two studies, only one of which was double-blinded and lasted six weeks. FDA approval of Risperdal for mania for children and adolescents aged 10–17 was granted based on one three-week double-blind trial. The high rates of dropout due to inefficacy and intolerability in the TEOSS follow-up study casts a large shadow of doubt on the clinical validity of these brief trials. Instead, disturbing facts are beginning to emerge over time as the realities of serious negative effects can no longer be spun and the real harm being wrought is uncovered in story after personal story.[23]

Considering the reality of meager improvements extracted from studies that utilize methodologies that favor finding treatment effects, weighed against consistent findings of significant adverse effects and largely untested long-term safety, a favorable risk/benefit profile in support of antipsychotics as first-line treatment for children and adolescents, regardless of the diagnosed disorder, appears untenable. The APA Working Group concurred, finding enough "significant risks" in its review to advise psychosocial treatments rather than antipsychotics for pediatric bipolar disorder (PBD), citing that nonpharmacological interventions "confer benefit with no risk".[24]

MYTH AND SCIENCE

When the evidence is explored, no reasonable scientist or practitioner would come down on the side of a favorable risk/benefit profile for pediatric use of antipsychotics. How, then, can we explain the fact that prescription rates continue their upward march in numbers and downward march in the age for which they are prescribed? How has it become so commonplace for antipsychotics to be listed first on the treatment plan for so many youth, even without manic or psychotic symptoms? The taken-for-granted acceptability and widespread use of pediatric antipsychotic drugs must be considered in light of the interests of those who have the most to gain. It is tempting to dismiss this viewpoint as cynical. We believe that not to explore a direction likely to shed light on the glaring discrepancy between the evidence and current practice is an ethical error on several counts. First, skeptical curiosity lies at the heart of the scientific and ethical enterprise—there should be no "Do Not Trespass" signs blocking the road. Second, scientific inquiry is critical. This does not mean that it points the finger like a critical teacher or parent, but it refuses to succumb to pressures to look away. Instead, critical science views restrictions on full exploration of the facts as indications that there likely are vested interests in diverting attention elsewhere. This possibility fuels the imperative even more to explore what those interests might be and how they operate. Finally, when it comes to safeguarding the rights and health of children, every road should be taken, particularly when common sense points the way and so much is at stake.

As a start on this path, we ask how our field has come to accept uncritically the proposition that many child and adolescent problems are not by-products of poverty, interpersonal distress, or other context-dependent factors, but of chronic disease and unbalanced neurotransmitters. We believe this collective myopia is *not* a triumph of science, but a triumph of marketing *over* science. It is, in short, a myth! Myths are stories, but bigger than your average fairy tale. They have the power to operate at basic, cultural levels and in unexamined ways.

That is, people don't identify their thoughts and actions as shaped by these "grand narratives";[25] they just act. In short, people live by myths without knowing it. The fact is, no one has identified any biological marker for any of the diagnosed conditions assigned to so many young people today.[26] Nevertheless, the *myth* of a biological foundation for certain childhood behaviors creates a certainty in which the prescription of powerful drugs for even the youngest and most vulnerable becomes automatic. And this is the breeding ground for decisions made by medical and nonmedical mental health practitioners.

Myths do not spring fully articulated overnight into the common consciousness but evolve over time. We suggest that the myth that children are well served by taking antipsychotic drugs has been constructed intentionally through the co-opting of science and media. It is not hard to see who might benefit from increased prescriptions. Psychiatric drugs comprise a hefty portion of the swelling drug sales in the United States. In 2009, antipsychotics maintained their number one ranking from 2008 as the top-selling class of drugs sold in the United States with $14.6 billion in sales.[27] Undoubtedly, the pharmaceutical industry is invested in the continued success of these highly profitable products.

One way to increase prescribing (and profit) is to offer financial incentives to physicians and psychiatrists in return for product promotion. For example, psychiatrists topped a recent published list of physicians receiving drug company money.[28] Payments to psychiatrists go for things like speaking fees, travel, meals, and consultation. Speakers' bureaus essentially turn physicians into mouthpieces for the industry. Psychiatrists give presentations, usually at upscale restaurants, using slides and responses to audience questions prepared by the drug manufacturer. Some argue that the largesse showered on physicians is legal and does not skew oaths to do no harm. However, physicians are susceptible to financial incentive as evidenced by increased prescription following pharmaceutical "perks."[29]

Pharmaceutical visits to prescribers not only include financial incentives but education to help busy doctors know the latest findings. Fortunately for the drug companies, the data is not hard to come by. Clinical drug trials are almost solely the purview of pharmaceutical companies who spend significant dollars to create networks of highly visible scientists to research their products. Invariably, the findings tell an optimistic story of the investigated drug's benefits, cloaked in the language of statistical and methodological intricacies. Can these stories be believed?

Unfortunately, what is pawned off to prescribers, medical and nonmedical mental health trainees, and the public is largely fiction. The notion that science is deliberately being manipulated to construct a particular tale cannot be simply chalked off as another conspiracy theory. The extent to which pharmaceutical companies have manipulated medical research for their own interests has been exposed by some of the most respected voices in the field. For example, Marcia Angell, former editor-in-chief of the *New England Journal of Medicine*, blew the whistle over a decade ago regarding the "ubiquitous and manifold . . . financial associations" authors of drug trials had to the companies whose drugs were being studied.[30] The editor-in-chief of the *Lancet* decried that "journals have devolved into information laundering operations for the pharmaceutical industry."[31] As yet another example, consider the recent exposé in the *New York Times* documenting drug company ghostwriting of an entire textbook for primary care physicians about recognition and treatment of psychiatric disorders.[32]

The result of industry influence is a direct correlation between who funds the study and its outcome. For example, in 2006 Heres looked at published comparative trials of five antipsychotic medications.[33] In 9 out of 10 studies, the drug made by the company that sponsored the trial was found to be superior. Davis, coauthor of the study, surmised that "90 percent of industry-sponsored studies that boast a prominent academic as the lead author are conducted by a company that later enlists a university researcher as the 'author'".[34] Similarly, *JAMA*'s systematic review found that "financial relationships among industry, scientific investigators, and academic institutions are pervasive," and "by combining data from articles examining 1140 studies, we found that industry-sponsored studies were significantly more likely to reach conclusions that were favorable to the sponsor than were non-industry studies".[35] Meanwhile, studies with negative findings for investigated drugs rarely see the light of print.[36] Angell, with more than a touch of sadness, concludes,

It is simply no longer possible to believe much of the clinical research that is' published, or to rely on the judgment of trusted physicians or authoritative medical guidelines. I take no pleasure in this conclusion, which I reached slowly and reluctantly over my two decades as an editor of *The New England Journal of Medicine*.[37]

Regarding pharmaceutical influence over the science of pediatric antipsychotics, one need not look far to detect a smoking gun. One highly visible researcher, Joseph Biederman, Harvard Medical School professor and psychiatrist at Massachusetts General Hospital, has touted the efficacy and safety of the antipsychotic Risperdal for more than a decade. From its early days as the drug of choice for children diagnosed with autism, Risperdal has migrated along with other potent antipsy-chotics to the popular pediatric bipolar diagnosis. This label has been so fervently championed by Biederman that reporter and historian Robert Whitaker has called him the "Pied Piper of pediatric bipolar disorder".[38] Thanks in large part to Biederman's efforts, PBD and anti-psychotics are now a taken-for-granted pairing.

As additional evidence of conflict of interest, an investigative report in the *New York Times* claimed that Biederman, in violation of Harvard policies, failed to report at least $1.4 million in income from drug com-panies.[39] A second article asserted that Biederman repeatedly asked Johnson & Johnson, makers of Risperdal, to fund a research center at Massachusetts General to focus on PBD.[40] A prime mission of the center, according to Biederman, would be to "move forward the com-mercial goals of J. & J." Johnson & Johnson allegedly joined with Bie-derman to produce science that favored Risperdal when Johnson & Johnson drafted a scientific abstract and requested Biederman's signa-ture. According to the report, the company also sought his advice on how to handle the fact that children given placebos in Risperdal trials also improved significantly. More recently, Senator Grassley of Iowa has broadened an investigation to learn if Biederman promised posi-tive results for Johnson & Johnson for studies yet to be conducted.[41]

Another researcher leading pediatric antipsychotic drug trials has significant connections to pharmaceuticals. Robert L. Findling, profes-sor of psychiatry and pediatrics at Case Western Reserve University and director of the Division of Child and Adolescent Psychiatry, Uni-versity Hospitals of Cleveland, is particularly visible as a contributor to a widely circulated online medical forum, Medscape. Findling serves as an advisor or consultant for 22 pharmaceutical companies, has served as a speaker or member of a speakers' bureau for 3, and has received research funding from 14.[42] Findling led the 2008 trial for aripiprazole (Abilify), a second-generation antipsychotic, for 13 to 17 year olds di-agnosed with schizophrenia.[43] Adolescents in the aripiprazole groups (10 mg and 30 mg) in this trial increased their body weight more than 5 percent, up to five times greater than youth in the placebo group. There were more than double as many youth experiencing extrapyra-midal disorder in the 10 milligram group and more than four times as many in the 30 milligram group compared with those in placebo. Abil-ify takers were as much as three times more likely to report somnolence than those on placebo. In spite of these glaring red flags, Findling con-cluded that Abilify was "generally well tolerated".[44]

One would hope that the pharmaceutical industry is kept in check through university ethics and government oversight. However, gov-ernment agencies and academic advisory panels, presumably the watchdogs over industry-sponsored research, are not the firewalls many would assume. Willman, in a Pulitzer Prize–winning report, found widespread breaches in ties of National Institutes of Health (NIH, umbrella organization of the NIMH) researchers to pharmaceutical money.[45] Whitaker has systematically detailed the involvement of the NIMH with industry propaganda promoting psychiatric products.[46] In addition, financial conflicts of interest among U.S. FDA advisory members are common.[47] Moreover, Cosgrove noted "strong financial ties between the industry and those responsible for developing . . . the diagnostic criteria for mental illness", especially where drugs are the first-line of treatment for a specified disorder.[48] Experts who formulate practice parameters often serve as consultants and speakers for major drug companies.[49] For example, the Texas Children's Medication Algorithm Project (TCMAP), funded by the Texas Department of State Health Services, convened a panel of experts to derive consensus-based recommendations for stepwise pediatric medication regimens (interestingly, of the higher priced drugs). Disclosure statements for prominent academics and researchers involved in TCMAP span nearly half an entire printed page.[50] Industry infiltration into all aspects of government-sponsored research, oversight regulation, and consensus panels means that clinicians and consumers have no safety net to fall back on for unbiased information and protection against the potential harm these drugs can cause the youngest in our society.

The net effect of drug industry control over psychiatric research is the construction of a distorted picture of actual risks and benefits of the drugs in question. Thus, clinicians and consumers weighing treatment options lack honest information to determine the best and most ethical course to pursue. It no longer can be assumed that time-honored journalistic peer-review or impartial government regulation produce a sound body of science to support ethical mental health practice. Clients and clinicians are essentially flying blind if they uncritically consume the cliff notes version of clinical trials to guide practice. Very few obstacles can withstand the onslaught of an industry as politically and financially powerful as the pharmaceuticals. They have ruthlessly violated long-standing rules of conduct for ethical research to enrich shareholders and perpetuate their wealth into the foreseeable future. In sum, science has been bought for corporate profit, even when it compromises the health of children who depend on adults for protection and who *are* the future.

MYTH AND MEDIA

It takes more than tainted science and drug reps to create myth. Myths are born when repeated, intersecting narratives converge over time into a unified superstory—in this case, one that permeates not only the halls of academia, the hospital, and public clinic, but also the classroom, the living room, and eventually the minds of whole populations within a culture. Like "Mom," "Apple Pie," and "Freedom for All," the superstory's unquestioned veracity does not permit the curtain to part on the multiple contradictions and darker sides that lie within it. In the case of our critical examination of antipsychotic medications for children, we can peer inside to see how this type of story comes about. What we find goes by the general term *media*, including print, television, and film as well as the various modes of electronic communication that occupy an immediate presence in the lives of so many. The long arm of the pharmaceutical industry is evident in all these, perhaps more than in the elite world of empirical research. Antonuccio, Danton, and McClanahan detail its reach beyond clinical trials—from Internet, direct-to consumer advertising, grassroots consumer advocacy, and professional guilds to medical schools and clinical training programs.[51] They conclude, "It is difficult to think of any arena involving information about medications that does not have significant industry financial or marketing influences".

Those involved in mental health practice, as members of the culture, take in all these forms of messaging, including professional press and the policies and procedures of work sites. For example, practice parameters for PBD approved by the American Academy of Child & Adolescent Psychiatry specifies pharmacotherapy as the minimal standard (applies 95% of the time or in almost all cases) for mania in bipolar I disorder for children.[52] Psychotherapy is considered to be adjunctive, relegated to teaching the child and caregivers about bipolar illness, including its heritability, and to ensure medication compliance. These so-called truths trickle down. The American Association of Marriage and Family Therapy (AAMFT) is a case in point. The AAMFT website describes "childhood-onset mental illness" (COMI) as "biologically based, meaning that chemicals or structures in the brain are not working as they are supposed to."[53] This means that "almost all children with bipolar disorders need to take medication to help stabilize their moods" and "many times, a combination of two or more medications works better, if one medication alone does not produce a satisfactory response."[54] This a striking testimony to the power of myth as the AAMFT represents a field founded on the belief that interpersonal dynamics more appropriately explain human distress than biology.

These types of unquestioned pronouncements are commonplace in many practice settings. For example, pharmaceutical intervention often is built in to mental health agency procedures via the psychiatrist who provides supervision and has prescribing power for more challenging cases. Pressure to think medical is established well before the first paid position and persists through the span of a career. For example, it is widely considered desirable to include *DSM* and psychopharmacology training in clinical graduate coursework, even in those fields most known for their emphasis on environmental influence. Trainees and experienced clinicians alike are inundated with invitations to workshops and continuing education courses so they can be up-to-date on the biology of the brain and the neurochemistry of psychotropics. Pharmacology and psychotherapy are rapidly aligning as inseparable, yet unequal, interventions in daily practice.

Having created and disseminated the science, the pharmaceutical/psychiatric conglomerate is in a position to define "do no harm" and set the terms of informed consent. Clinicians choosing nonmedical options may fear the risk of a lawsuit and even censure from their own peers and professional guilds for ignoring science and practicing unethically. In so many ways, the psychiatric establishment enshrines psychopharmacology as best *and* ethical practice.[55]

How many stories are told, in one form or another, of the out-of-control, defiant child destined to fail at school and wind up behind bars, magically transformed into an obedient, studious youngster with the help of a pill. How many parents would want to deny their child the chance to star in this story? And how many clinicians would not want the same for their young clients? Bleeding through these trouble-to-triumph narratives are those that speak about irreversible tremors, life-shortening obesity, or a child's death at the hands of a potent psychiatric drug cocktail. In spite of counterstories, the view that antipsychotics *must* be given and are reasonably safe for children exhibiting certain forms of extreme behavior has become accepted and normal.

CRITICAL ETHICS

This is the world in which medical and nonmedical mental health professionals live and practice. It is a world where certain child behaviors are assumed to be heritable, organically based diseases and where subduing difficult and aggressive youths is ethically justified by a belief that such treatment wards off a future life as a social outcast or degenerate. The mandate of medical intervention imposed by a dominant medical paradigm hangs over the head of the nonmedical practitioner. With the presumption of science behind it, the most evident ethical choice is to defer to medical expertise. In the world of everyday practice, this means that psychologists, social workers, and other mental health clinicians refer their most troubled youngsters for psychiatric evaluation. And, psychiatric evaluation almost always includes medication. Psychotherapists, then, are left to police the medical regimen and mitigate the fallout of the disorder in the child's world. Psychologists and mental health professionals cannot—*are not qualified to*—treat the underlying disorder.

In such a world, how can a practicing, nonmedical mental health clinician respond when faced with the immediate crisis of a child out of control, at risk of self-harm, or inexplicably exhibiting strange or frightening behaviors? Is the most ethical action one that follows the treatment guidelines constructed by the financial and political clout of a for-profit industry linked to the psychiatric establishment? Or, is the most ethical choice one that is based on a critical examination of the science, including knowledge of one's own ability to provide effective, nonpharmacological help and an awareness of context (e.g., cultural, socioeconomic, racial, gender, and sexual orientation disparities) that expands understanding of presented problems in terms other than discreet psychiatric disorders and biology? It is likely no surprise at this point that we believe that critical analysis lies at the heart of ethical practice. Without it, do no harm and informed consent are largely preset by entities whose ethics may serve the well-being of stockholders rather than children.

Critical ethics does not stop, however, with critical analysis but requires practitioners to advocate for greater transparency in research and the dissemination of critical commentary into the public sphere. It also urges practitioners to become advocates for change within their practice and professional circles. Further, consistent with standing mental health ethical mandates, critical ethics obligates clinicians, within the scope of their expertise, to act for the betterment of client welfare and to provide information regarding the risks of their treatment. It is our view that it is within the scope of nonmedical clinicians' expertise to provide counseling and psychological intervention for problems facing children frequently considered biological in origin. Moreover, this intervention is justifiable as primary and standalone, rather than merely adjunctive, based on the client's preference. In addition, nonmedical practitioners have a right and obligation to share reasonable and researched information about the risks and benefits of psychiatric medications with their clients when this is a relevant concern for the client. This information falls within the range of expected knowledge for any practitioner today and requires that he or she be informed beyond drug company propaganda. To threaten clinicians under the guise of ethics violation when they provide information regarding known drug risks undermines their right to assist clients making critical decisions about treatment. Furthermore, it begs the question of why nonmedical clinicians are asked to become fluent in psychopharmacology so that pharmacological intervention can be suggested for an ever-expanding range of child difficulties but are forbidden to seek and use knowledge to offer a more research-based picture. Our concept of critical ethics, therefore, requires that mental health clinicians, consistent with their code of ethics, take the following steps[56]:

1. *Become educated in how to evaluate research for methodological flaws, bias, and conflicts of interest, and discern noteworthy, underreported findings.* Research needs to be studied in its originally published form with a careful exploration of flaws and conflicts of interest.[57]

2. *Become educated about the evidence base for nonpharmacological interventions.* Clinicians should have a solid knowledge of nonmedical options for the variety of problem behaviors they might encounter in their client population. Moreover, they should have confidence that these approaches have proven records of efficacy and are powerful, no-risk forces for positive change.[58]

3. *Hold a questioning attitude regarding media portrayals of psychotropic medications for children.* Practitioners need to be wary of slick websites and know how to find out who produces or sanctions their content and provides funding. If it sounds too rosy or too cozy to be true, it probably is.

4. *Provide true informed consent to clients, including informing clients of the risks and benefits of antipsychotic medications for children and adolescents.* In providing real informed consent, children, even those of school age or younger, and their parents and/or caregivers need to know the meaning of off-label prescription, the lack of evidence for acute and long-term antipsychotic pediatric use, and the real risks these drugs entail. The fact that children are not legally able to give consent, but rely on parents or caretakers to act in their best interest, should not deter clinicians from gaining youth assent. It is ethically justified, and empirically supported, to elicit and address children's questions and concerns, especially when it involves psychiatric medications that are likely to profoundly influence a child's day-to-day life as well as future. Given a young person's dependent status on adults underscores the ethical imperative that clinicians give balanced information to caretakers who ultimately will make the final call regarding their child's treatment.[59]

5. *Support clients to be at the helm of their treatment, regardless of the choice to take or not take psychotropic medications.* At each step, children and caregivers' preferences are honored. If antipsychotic medications are chosen, clinicians can help the youth and parents/ caregivers be in the driver's seat, to monitor side effects or to decide when to discontinue the drugs. All too often, the prestige of prescribing physicians or psychiatrists intimidates consumers and stifles their questions and preferences. Systematically obtaining regular feedback from all involved, including the young person and caregivers, helps ensure that their preferences are privileged throughout treatment.[60]

6. *Help children, adolescents, and their caregivers become critical consumers.* For clients who want to know more, clinicians can inform them that much of what can be

found on the Internet is biased and urge them to seek information from a variety of reputable and unbiased sources, including psychiatrists or physicians, before committing to a particular treatment.

7. *Work for change in mental health agencies, organizations, and institutions to combat the appropriation of mental health counseling and psychotherapy by medical, for-profit enterprises.* Working ethically, one client at a time is essential, but not enough. Without taking a stand for transparency and change beyond the immediate level of therapeutic practice, we are part of the problem. The larger structures in place at every level of mental health—funding, policies, procedures, and training, for example—ensure that the business of mental health operates in specific ways. In child and adolescent mental health, these structures, for the most part, promote medical intervention. Change at these levels does not occur solely within the therapeutic encounter, but in the professional and public sphere through direct challenge and proposal of alternative discourses. This additional step means that we advocate for a transformation of our professions for the welfare of our clients and as reclamation of our identity as helpers.[61]

ETHICS IN ACTION

Science, in the case of childhood psychiatric drugs, is not the objective, pure, and noble enterprise that holds such sway in the popular imagination. The dark cloud of corruption hangs over it in the form of multiple and enduring financial ties to industry whose primary purpose is to increase profit. Tainted science is not an ethical foundation upon which to base any practice designed to serve the welfare of the public, much less the youngest in our society who count on us for protection. The ethics we propose is critical in that it looks beneath the veneer of myth to discern meaningful scientific evidence. It is critical also in the sense that it provides an important safeguard for maintaining the independence and integrity of the work most of us chose because of our desire to be of help to others.[62]

Critical ethics requires time and energy. It is much easier to take the common wisdom at face value and go on with one's practice and life. Our belief is that this constitutes a violation of the ethical imperative that we do no harm to our clients and that we provide them with genuine informed consent. Even more than time and energy, critical ethics requires courage. This means courage to do no harm after you know what you know, despite possible repercussions. It means the courage to act locally in one's workplace or professional group to challenge unquestioned assumptions. For example, it is an act of great courage to simply question, in the midst of the staff meeting with the psychiatrist, the validity and usefulness of a child's diagnosis of bipolar disorder or the prescription of more than one drug.

Finally, critical ethics means reclaiming one's identity as a helper, not just for those worrisome, expected problems, but for young people and their families in dire distress. If we cannot be of help to those who come to us, is it ethical for us to practice at all? For example, several meetings with the mother and her daughter, Alison, who had cut her arms, meant that many aspects of their lives became relevant to the presenting problem, not just the more visible act of cutting. In the first session, the mother listened with astonishment as her daughter mentioned that she had read about cutting in a teen magazine and thought it might help her feel better after the breakup with her boyfriend. To everyone's relief, she proclaimed that it only made things worse and vowed not to try it again. What had started out as a possible trip to the emergency room turned into a routine (if these discussions are ever routine) heart-to-heart talk between mother and daughter, with the clinician as referee, about the daughter's privacy and her desire for a later curfew. In the context of no other identifiable risk factors in her life, including normative scores on the intake psychological assessment and the obvious presence of a watchful and caring mother, this family avoided the march toward medication and resolved a crisis of adolescent development over the course of a few meetings. The strong relationship the clinician established with Alison and her mother reassured the clinician, that, if there were additional signs of danger, the family would seek his help.

Similarly, the young boy, Nathan, who sought safety at the top of the school flagpole, after being coaxed down, found the open arms and ears of teachers, his social worker, and a home-based counselor where he talked mostly about the recent passing of his father and the trouble he was having in his new foster home. When asked what he needed, he listed two things—his bicycle (stored at a relative's home in another city) and a chance to be reunited with his two sisters, even if for a day. These wishes clearly did not require medications, nor could they be found in any standard book of psychological techniques. However, retrieving the bike as first order of business showed this young boy that people took him seriously and gave him a sense of normalcy and an important vehicle, literally, to make friends in his new neighborhood. A trip to spend the day at the ocean allowed the siblings to be together, to see that each was okay, and to share their memories about that fateful Christmas Eve when their father, the rock of their struggling, single-parent family, died suddenly. Over the course of the next six months, a plan was created for a permanent home for Nathan, one that included regular contact with his siblings. Nathan settled into his schoolwork and graduated on time with his class.

Finally, for Kyle, the tantrum-prone five-year old, the solution was standard parenting management strategies combined with a reevaluation of how the father's job and the family's finances meant that Kyle's mother shouldered the burden of parenting for Kyle as well as his little sister. When the family established more shared parenting and more fun time together, Kyle's behavior improved dramatically.

Nathan's case was time intensive and involved a whole team of helpers, whereas only one therapist and several meetings were needed to help Alison get her life back on track. Work with Kyle and his family involved eight family meetings and collaboration with his preschool teacher. All three cases required empirically informed skills. This is the everyday work of mental health professionals that is far from ordinary and far from second rate. It challenges the view of the necessity of powerful antipsychotics for so many of the problems faced by children and their families arriving at the doorstep of our offices. This is the work of the critical ethical practitioner.

6

Legal Issues Surrounding the Psychiatric Drugging of Children and Youth

Jim Gottstein

INTRODUCTION

When I read Robert Whitaker's *Mad in America,* I realized it was not only an incisive book about our misguided and harmful mental health system, but also, potentially a litigation road map to challenge forced psychiatric drugging. As a lawyer who narrowly escaped becoming a permanent mental patient as a result of psychiatric treatment, I felt I was in a unique position to tackle this issue. In 2002, I cofounded the Law Project for Psychiatric Rights (PsychRights) with Don Roberts and Chris Cyphers to mount a strategic litigation campaign against forced psychiatric drugging and electroshock. We started out with a focus on the forced drugging of adults, but when we saw that what was happening to children and youth was even more horrific, we decided we had to make them our priority. Since children are almost always *forced* to take psychiatric drugs by the adults in control of their lives, addressing this problem certainly fit within PsychRights' mission.

Children and youth on Medicaid are four times more likely to be given neuroleptics than those with private insurance. Neuroleptics are often referred to as antipsychotics, but since they have little, if any, antipsychotic properties, I use the word neuroleptic instead. Neuroleptic was the word originally given to this class of drugs, and means "seize the brain." They also used to be called major tranquilizers, to distinguish them from the benzodiazepines, such as Valium, which were referred to as minor tranquilizers. The word antipsychotic is marketing hype, pure and simple.

Parents of children on Medicaid whose boisterous, unruly, or disobedient behavior is challenging for their teachers are often informed by school officials that their children will not be allowed to continue in school unless they take psychiatric drugs. A medication demand may ensue just from that, or the child might be sent for a mental health evaluation that results in a prescription. Even more troubling is the increasingly prevalent mental health screening, which Gwen Olsen discussed in chapter 4. Mental health screening programs such as Teen Screen appear at face value to be government-sponsored programs designed to heighten awareness about childhood mental illness and to facilitate early intervention. In fact, they are developed and funded by drug companies to encourage a higher volume of psychiatric diagnoses and drug sales. The screenings are notorious for generating very high false positives. In other words, mental health screening is a "Drugging Dragnet."

If parents don't comply with drugging recommendations, schools often prohibit their child from attending. Worse still, parents are sometimes accused of neglecting the medical needs of their child and threatened by child protection agencies that their child will be taken away from them if they don't comply. This type of threat is often carried out. In summary, parents are forced to make their children take psychiatric drugs or risk their expulsion from school and even loss of custody. And God help children and youth in foster care, who have been taken away from their parents. While even parents living in poverty and relying on Medicaid can sometimes stand up for their children's rights, once the government has seized them, they are virtually powerless to stop them from being drugged. I have been involved with a group of foster youth and former foster youth called Facing Foster Care in Alaska since 2008, and when I ask these youth and alumni how many have been given psychiatric drugs, almost all of them answer in the affirmative.

From a lawyer's perspective, the overwhelming amount of harm being done to children and youth through psychiatric drugging, especially by the neuroleptics, raises a host of legal questions. For example, what are the responsibilities of non-MD mental health specialists such as psychologists and social workers in light of the fact that neuroleptic drugs rarely help children and cause great harm? Can psychologists tell their clients these truths when their MD is telling them something else? Must they? Can psychologists challenge a psychiatrist's diagnosis? What legal rights do children and youth have to be protected from the harm caused by psychiatric drugs? What legal approaches might be taken to address the problem? What legal efforts have already been taken? What legal efforts can parents, mental health professionals, and others concerned about these issues initiate or join?

TRUTH-TELLING OBLIGATIONS OF MENTAL HEALTH PROFESSIONALS

Psychologists, psychiatrists, and social workers have codes of ethics that have varying requirements regarding being faithful to science and the truth.[1]

Section 2 of the American Medical Association's Principles of Medical Ethics states that physicians, including psychiatrists, have an absolute obligation of truth telling and to expose those who are not telling the truth. So what flows from this? At the very least, psychiatrists and other physicians prescribing neuroleptics have an obligation to inform parents and older children of the adverse effects and risks, and to let them know when they are prescribing neuroleptics in ways that are not FDA approved (as a sleep aid, for example). As a society, we have placed our trust in the medical profession to objectively evaluate possible treatments and not be swayed by the false marketing of drug companies. Physicians prescribing neuroleptics to children and youth are betraying that trust. It is precisely this betrayal of trust that obligates those in other mental health professions who care about children and youth to protect them from the harm caused by neuroleptics.

Psychologists, under their code of ethics, are obligated to (a) do no harm; (b) promote accuracy, honesty, and truthfulness; (c) not . . . engage in fraud, subterfuge, or intentional misrepresentation of fact; (d) take reasonable steps to avoid harming their clients/patients; and (e) base their work on established scientific and professional knowledge.

Conflicts between Ethics and Organizational Demands

As Sparks and Duncan discuss in chapter 5, the 2006 report of the American Psychological Association (APA) Working Group on Psychoactive Medications for Children and Adolescents was highly critical of the widespread use of neuroleptic medications. However, the APA's Code of Ethics also has the following provision:

If the demands of an organization with which psychologists are affiliated or for whom they are working conflict with this Ethics Code, psychologists clarify the nature of the conflict, make known their commitment to the Ethics Code, and to the extent feasible, resolve the conflict in a way that permits adherence to the Ethics Code.

This means that they only have to comply with their code of ethics when it conflicts with their organizational demands, if it is "feasible." That psychologists are allowed to violate their ethical principles because it is part of their job is shocking, but it doesn't excuse them from the *moral* obligation to do no harm. The United Nations' Special Rapporteur on torture and other cruel, inhuman, or degrading treatment or punishment has concluded that giving people neuroleptics against their will can constitute torture,[2] and the APA has adopted the position that it is never acceptable to participate in torture.[3] As such, psychologists may very well be violating their ethical responsibilities by participating in the practice of prescribing children and youth neuroleptics.

As several authors have already discussed, the diagnosis of pediatric bipolar disorder has been heavily promoted by the pharmaceutical industry over the last 20 years for the express purpose of creating a child market for neuroleptics, branded as *antipsychotics* and *mood stabilizers.* Drug companies have achieved these goals by financing key opinion leaders in psychiatry to extol the virtues of these drugs while denying their dangers, publishing fraudulent ghostwritten articles in prestigious journals and unleashing armies of sales representatives to convince doctors to prescribe them for an ever-increasing list of childhood conditions.

Since it is the diagnosis that justifies the drugging, it is critically important that children and youth not be improperly diagnosed with a mental disorder that results in a neuroleptic prescription. Licensed psychologists are independent practitioners who have the mandate to diagnose within their areas of training and expertise. Psychologists therefore have the right and responsibility to change a diagnosis if they believe that their client was wrongfully diagnosed by another mental health professional. And it goes without saying that if they believe a child's behavior, as trying as it might be for teachers or parents, doesn't warrant a diagnosis, they have a responsibility to convey this as well. Some psychologists, especially those who work in institutions headed by psychiatrists, may feel that challenging a psychiatrist's diagnosis renders them vulnerable to accusations that they are engaging in the unauthorized practice of medicine. It is not the unauthorized practice of medicine if it is the authorized practice of psychology. For example, the following provision is from Washington State statutes: "The prohibition on the unauthorized practice of medicine does not prohibit the practice of any healing art for which the practitioner is licensed."[4]

In addition to challenging incorrect diagnoses, psychologists treating children who are taking psychiatric drugs have the right and responsibility to inquire whether the prescribing physician informed the parents of the side effects and long-term ramifications of the medication their child is taking, and whether they are aware of evidence-based psychosocial approaches, several of which are discussed in chapters 7 through 10. Psychologists who work with children whose diagnoses are typically treated with medication have a responsibility to keep up with the literature on those medications.

Sharing information with parents about the medication that their children are taking also leads some psychologists to feel vulnerable to the accusation of "practicing medicine without a license." When for example, a psychologist discovers that a pediatrician who has no formal mental health training has casually prescribed a neuroleptic for reasons that are not even FDA approved and hasn't informed the family of the risks involved, it is ironic that it is the psychologist rather than the MD who feels vulnerable to the charge of malpractice.

In spite of these fears, I found virtually no cases in which psychologists were actually charged with the unauthorized practice of medicine, which suggests the problem is theoretical. One case I did find, *Wesley v. Greyhound Lines, Inc.*, held that a psychologist rendering psychological services as defined under state law was not engaged in the unauthorized practice of medicine even though psychologists were not specifically exempted from the statute defining the unauthorized practice of medicine.[5] In other words, the *Wesley* case applies the general principle that the licensed practice of a healing art, such as psychology, as set forth in the Washington statute, is not the unauthorized practice of medicine.

The bottom line is that psychologists who advise patients and their families about neuroleptics are not very likely to be accused of engaging in the unauthorized practice of medicine so long as it is the authorized practice of psychology. It is critical that psychologists be a voice for truth by informing the children and families in their care that neuroleptics are extremely harmful and there is no valid evidence that they are helpful, as has been amply documented by Whitaker in chapter 1 and by Sparks and Duncan in chapter 5.

In contrast to the psychologists' code of ethics, the social workers' code of ethics not only requires them to act honestly and responsibly, but also to promote ethical practices on the part of their employers. In addition, social workers are required to critically examine and keep current with emerging knowledge and are not allowed to participate in, condone, or be associated with dishonesty fraud, or deception.[6]

While the specific details of their licensing and roles may be somewhat different, the same basic analysis should also hold true for social workers. Thus, when acting within the scope of their practice, social workers should also inform children and their families with whom they are working about the truth, namely, that neuroleptics are extremely harmful and there is no valid evidence that they are helpful. Social workers should also make their view known to the general public regarding the truth about psychiatric drugs.

When consulted, psychologists, social workers, and other mental health professionals should inform clients not only about the harms of neuroleptic drugs, but also about evidence-based approaches to treatment that don't involve drugs, and that they routinely use in their own practices but are less well known to the general public.

The CriticalThinkRx.org curriculum is a compendium of evidence-based, effective nondrug approaches to mental health care for children and youth.[7] CriticalThinkRx was paid for by a grant from the Attorneys General Consumer and Prescriber Grant Program, funded by the multistate settlement of consumer fraud claims regarding the illegal marketing of Neurontin. CriticalThinkRx was developed specifically for nonmedical personnel working with children who have been prescribed or are likely to be prescribed psychiatric drugs. It is an authoritative program on the use of psychiatric drugs with children that describes evidence-based psychosocial approaches with children and youth. It was created for the express purpose of enabling mental health professionals such as psychologists, social workers, school psychologists, and juvenile justice and child protection personnel to make informed decisions on behalf of the children in their care. It can also be of tremendous help to parents trying to keep their children from being drugged by the state. The CriticalThinkRx website address is http://criticalthinkrx.org/.

To summarize, psychologists, social workers, and other mental health professionals have an obligation to do what they can to stop the carnage caused by the use of neuroleptics on children and youth. This involves truth telling about the harm caused by, and lack of effectiveness of, the neuroleptics; reversing improper diagnoses when appropriate; and informing clients about, and utilizing, the many nondrug approaches that have been proved to be helpful without causing harm.

RIGHTS OF CHILDREN AND YOUTH NOT TO BE HARMED BY PSYCHIATRIC DRUGS

Since neuroleptics are so harmful to children and youth with no counterbalancing benefit, the question naturally arises, What rights do children and youth have to be protected from these drugs?

U.S. Constitutional Law

Children and youth in state custody such as the juvenile justice system and foster care have the constitutional right not to be harmed by psychotropic drugs through government action or inaction. In 1989, the U.S. Supreme Court held in the *Deshaney* case that a state did not violate the U.S. Constitution when it discharged a child into the custody of an abusive father, but, when the state takes a person into its custody and holds him there against his will, the Constitution imposes upon it a corresponding duty to assume some responsibility for his safety and general well-being. The rationale for this principle is simple enough: when the state by the affirmative exercise of its power so restrains an individual's liberty that it renders him unable to care for himself, and at the same time fails to provide for his basic human needs—for example, food, clothing, shelter, medical care, and reasonable safety—it transgresses the substantive limits on state action set by the Eighth Amendment and the due process clause.[8]

As is graphically demonstrated by Robert Whitaker in chapter 1, neuroleptics cause extreme harm to children with little or no benefit. Thus, at least in my view, *Deshaney* confirms that children and youth have the right under the U.S. Constitution to be protected from these harms when in state custody. This raises the question of whether these rights may only be enforced by parents, or whether children and youth may enforce these rights on their own behalf. While I have not seen any published case directly addressing this question, under the same type of analysis used for other constitutional rights, the answer seems to be yes, children do have substantial rights to try to enforce their own constitutional rights.[9]

State Law

Presumably, most if not all state constitutions afford protection similar to that under the U.S. Constitution pursuant to *Deshaney*. At least some states, such as New Jersey, California, Alaska, and Florida, also recognize that children and youth can assert such state constitutional rights on their own behalf, although such enforcement rights are not as extensive as for adults.[10] Thus, both children and parents can assert the child's right to be protected from neuroleptics while in state custody. In addition, according to attorney Rachel Camp, "many states include a version of the following in their statutory definition of legal custody: the right to have physical possession of the child; the right and duty to protect, train, and discipline the child; and the responsibility to provide the child with food, clothing, shelter, and education."[11]

These rights tend to be fairly well defined in statutes and regulations, but with respect to being free of the administration of psychotropic drugs at least, such rights are regularly ignored. For example, in many, if not most states, unless their rights have been terminated, parents still have the right to give or withhold consent for psychotropic drugs. The reality, however, is that parents are frequently subject to co-ercion when being asked for such consent. This includes being threat-ened with termination of their parental rights, ending any possibility of reunification or having contact with their children. At other times, the requirement for parental consent is simply ignored. I know of in-stances where parents' children have been taken away from them be-cause they refuse to consent to the use of psychiatric drugs.

One such case took place in Detroit in March 2011. Maryanne God-boldo took her 13-year-old daughter Ariana to a children's clinic as-sociated with Child Protective Services (CPS) after she developed behavioral problems following a series of immunization shots in 2010. After a very brief evaluation at the clinic, Ariana was prescribed a neuroleptic. Ariana's symptoms only worsened, and Ms. Godboldo decided to consult another psychiatrist who felt that it was in Ariana's best interest to be weaned from the medication. When Ms. Godboldo told a therapist at the clinic that her daughter was no longer taking her neuroleptic drugs, the therapist reported her to CPS, accusing Ms. Godboldo of neglecting her daughter by failing to give her the medication in spite of the fact that Ms. Godboldo had consulted with and followed the advice of another physician. When Ms. Godboldo refused to comply with CPS demands, CPS workers showed up at her house with the police, who said they had a warrant to take the child. However, according to Ms. Godboldo's lawyer, Wanda Evans, officers never produced a warrant even after Ms. Godboldo repeat-edly asked to see it. A standoff ensued. A gunshot was reportedly fired from inside when the police started breaking into her house—though, according to Evans, not at officers. Finally, after long hours of tense negotiations, Ms. Godboldo—a mother, teacher, dancer, and respected figure in the city's arts circles—surrendered and was jailed and charged with multiple felony charges, and her daughter was placed in foster care.[12]

Because the community rallied around Ms. Godboldo and her daughter, and because Ms. Godboldo has effective legal representa-tion, as of this writing, she has been released from jail on bail. Ariana has not been drugged, because she is doing well off the drugs and was later released to a family member. However, as of this writing, final custody is still in question, and felony criminal charges are still pend-ing against Ms. Godboldo. One of the legal issues in the case is whether there was actually a valid court order because the one that CPS was fi-nally forced to produce appears to have been rubber stamped by CPS, not signed by the judge, and it is internally inconsistent. There is a website with information on Maryanne and Ariana, which publishes updates as they occur at http://www.justice4maryanne.com/.

The explanation given for seizing children in these circumstances is that the parents are neglecting the medical needs of their children by denying them psychiatric drugs. At this point, the reader is fully aware of how harmful neuroleptics are to children and the lengths to which the pharmaceutical industry will go to create and promote new diagnoses in order to market their drugs. Unfortunately, though, judges are swayed by this argument because with unlimited funds at their disposal, drug companies have created a belief system that permeates the culture, and there is no effective legal opposition to the state's application to seize the child.

Once a child has been seized by the state, with rare, if any, exceptions, the legal standard for when a child may be given psychotropic drugs is whether it is in their best interests. In a recent case, the District of Columbia Court of Appeals specifically ruled that (1) the child protective agency does not have authority to consent to psychotropic drugs, (2) the trial court does not have the authority to direct the child protection agency to make the decision, (3) the trial court has to make such a decision to override a parent's refusal to consent, and (4) the trial court must find by clear and convincing evidence that administering psychotropic drugs(s) would be in the best interests of the child.[13] This last principle is extremely important because, as other chapters in this book conclusively demonstrate, neuroleptics are rarely, if ever, in the best interests of children.*

The challenge is not establishing children's legal rights to be protected from neuroleptics. Rather it is enforcing these rights because most people in these situations do not have the resources to obtain good legal representation. Parents are often entitled to an attorney at state expense, and children often have a person appointed to represent their separate interests, called a *guardian ad litem,* who is supposed to make an *independent* investigation and advise the court as to the best interests of the child in the litigation. Unfortunately, such representation is usually lackluster at best, and these state-paid advocates do not truly represent the interests of the child. In other words, these state-paid advocates tend not to challenge the state's proposed action, making a sham of the legal proceedings. Obtaining a zealous advocate who truly represents the parent and child and who is knowledgeable about psychotropic drugs is extremely difficult in the current legal framework. If such advocates were available to present vigorous defenses

---

* It also seems that children and youth have the right to be protected from the harm caused by neuroleptics even when their parents or guardians choose to give them, but this is a far harder case to make, and the most pervasive abuses are inflicted upon children and youth in state custody.

at the trial-court level, prosecute appeals, and seek delays while appeals are pending, most of the psychiatric drugging of children in state custody would not occur. At the same time, a parent who resists the pressure can often be successful. The Ariana and Maryanne Godboldo situation illustrates this point. It is because the community rallied around Ms. Godboldo that she is receiving zealous legal representation, and media scrutiny is making all the difference in the world.

International Law

Associate Professor Angela Burton at New York School of Law, City University presents a compelling case in her recent law review article that the way in which children and youth are given psychotropic drugs in the United States violates international law.[14] The United States is a signatory to the 1971 United Nations Convention on Psychotropic Substances (1971 Convention), which, among other things, (1) requires that the use of psychotropic drugs is strictly limited to medical and scientific purposes and (2) prohibits advertising of psychotropic drugs to the general public with due regard to constitutional provisions. Chapter 1 makes it abundantly clear that science does not support the use of neuroleptic drugs for children. In fact, the vast majority of neuroleptic prescriptions to children are for indications for which the FDA has not granted approval, nor is their use supported by recognized medical references. Furthermore, direct-to-consumer, ask-your-doctor advertising has dramatically increased psychiatric drug use among children.

The United States is alone among recognized countries in refusing to ratify the United Nations Convention on the Rights of the Child (Child Rights Convention). However, it may very well be that under the Vienna Convention, as well as "customary international law," the United States is obligated to comply with the Child Rights Convention unless and until the Senate votes to reject it.[15] The central principle of the Child Rights Convention is "the best interests of the child shall be a primary consideration" for any government action regarding the child, including the obligation to ensure that institutions comply.[16] The most fundamental requirement for the implementation of the Child Rights Convention is that the child is recognized and fully respected as a human being with rights.[17] The Child Rights Convention is the first international document to give children full rights, independent of their parents.[18] As other chapters amply demonstrate, the vast majority of neuroleptic drug prescriptions to children in state custody cannot meet these international requirements.

REMEDIES

A right without a remedy is no right at all in any practical sense, so it is important to identify specific legal efforts that might be undertaken to enforce children's and youths' rights to be protected from neuroleptics.

Declaratory and Injunctive Relief

The most direct challenge is to seek a ruling from the court that children and youth have the right to be protected from harmful psychiatric drugging, combined with an injunction to prohibit the state from doing so. Just such a case was filed in September of 2008 against the state of Alaska by PsychRights, asking that Alaskan children and youth on Medicaid or in state custody be protected from being given psychotropic drugs unless and until:

(i)   evidence-based psychosocial interventions have been exhausted

(ii) the rationally anticipated benefits of psychotropic drug treatment outweigh the risks

(iii) the person or entity authorizing administration of the drug(s) is fully informed

(iv) close monitoring of, and appropriate means of responding to, treatment emergent effects are in place

(v)   all children and youth currently receiving such drugs be evaluated and brought into compliance with the above

PsychRights v. Alaska[19] was substantially based on the CriticalThinkRx.org curriculum,[20] which provides the evidence to support a significant reduction in the use of psychotropic drugs with children and youth. In addition to asserting the constitutional right to be protected from the harm caused by psychiatric drugs, *PsychRights v. Alaska* asserted that under state statutes, the state and its agents have a duty to care for the emotional, mental, and social needs of the child. This includes providing protection, nurture, training, discipline, education, medical care, as well as habilitative and rehabilitative treatment and services for children and youth diagnosed with a mental illness.[21] Ultimately, the Alaska Supreme Court ruled PsychRights did not have *standing*, which means the right to bring the lawsuit, because it was not personally harmed by the psychiatric drugging of children and youth. When the lawsuit was filed, the law was clear that PsychRights had the right to bring the case under Alaska's then expansive rules on the right to sue. These rules allowed a citizen-taxpayer to bring suit when the matter is of public importance and there is no more appropriate plaintiff that has or is likely to bring suit. However, the Alaska Supreme Court has been restricting such rights of citizen-taxpayers since *PsychRights v. Alaska* was filed, resulting in the dismissal of *PsychRights v. Alaska*.

The Court did state that a new case could be filed by a parent, but the short shrift the Alaska Supreme Court gave to the grave problem of protecting children and youth from psychiatric drugs while ignoring the other important reasons PsychRights brought the case in its own name, including the severe retaliation and possibility of legal fees being imposed on a parent bringing such a suit, has led PsychRights to look for other avenues.

Federal Civil Rights Action (42 U.S.C. & 1983)

There is a Civil War–era civil rights statute, commonly referred to as "§ 1983," that allows citizens to bring suit in federal court against people acting "under color of state law" for violations of the U.S. Constitution and laws.[22] Acting under color of state law essentially means utilizing state authority. An example is when a case worker for a child protection agency seizes a child and puts him or her in foster care. Another example is when foster parents give psychiatric drugs to their foster children. In both cases, state action is present because their authority derives from the state's power. Damages (money) and injunctions are available under §1983.

As of this writing, PsychRights is evaluating whether to refile a *PsychRights v. Alaska* type of case in federal court under § 1983. Inclusion of claims based on state law claim may or may not be allowed, and it would only apply to children and youth in state custody, whereas *PsychRights v. Alaska* also applied to children and youth on Medicaid who were not in state custody. Even without claims based on state law, a § 1983 case could be a very powerful way to address the problem. In addition to asserting the *Deshaney* right to be protected from harm while in state custody, rights under the Child Rights Convention and the 1971 Convention might also be asserted.

International Law

It is also possible to directly file a petition to an international tribunal for enforcement of the 1971 Convention. It is less clear whether such a petition could be filed under the Child Rights Convention since it has not been ratified by the Senate. As a practical matter, such petitions would likely be primarily symbolic. This is not necessarily a bad thing.

Medicaid Fraud/False Claims Act

Children living in poverty are given psychiatric drugs at a much higher rate than children of more affluent, empowered parents. Worse still, up to 50 percent of children and youth in foster care on any given day are on psychiatric drugs.[23] Medicaid is paying for most of these drugs in spite of the fact that in a majority of cases children are prescribed neuroleptics off label. Congress expressly prohibits Medicaid from paying for off-label prescriptions unless it is for a condition that is "supported" by at least one of three specified drug references referred to as *compendia,* which is called a "medically accepted indication."[24] PsychRights has developed a list of common psychiatric drugs prescribed to children and youth, identifying which diagnoses are allowable for which outpatient drugs under Medicaid for anyone under 18.[25] For example, there is no medically accepted indication for the use of the neuroleptic Geodon for anyone under the age of 18. Thus, any prescription of Geodon to a Medicaid recipient under 18 is fraudulent. Another example is that Seroquel is often prescribed for sleep. This is not a medically accepted indication, and it is therefore fraudulent when such a prescription is submitted to Medicaid.

Under the federal False Claims Act, anyone with information about Medicaid fraud that has not been "publicly disclosed" as defined in the act under the "Public Disclosure Bar," can bring a lawsuit in federal court for the fraud and share in the recovery, if any.[26] Under the False Claims Act: It is a false claim to knowingly present, or cause to be presented, a false or fraudulent claim for payment or approval to the federal government.[27] *Knowingly* is defined as (i) actual knowledge, (ii) deliberate ignorance of the truth or falsity, or (iii) reckless disregard of the truth or falsity, and no proof of intent to defraud is required.[28]

Every Medicaid provider is presumed to know what Medicaid's billing and coverage policies require.[29] A claim of ignorance is no excuse for doctors' failure to live up to their duty to familiarize themselves with the Medicaid requirements and observe their legal duty to submit authorized claims.[30] The rules about what *public disclosure* means is the subject of a lot of litigation. However, it is PsychRights' position that identification of specific prescriptions submitted to Medicaid is sufficient to get past the Public Disclosure Bar so long as those prescriptions are themselves not public. This is currently a hotly contested issue.

Cases under the False Claims Act are often called *whistleblower* cases, or *qui tam* actions, meaning these cases are brought on behalf of the government. Each offending prescription carries a minimum penalty of $5,500. These cases have a lot of other technical requirements, and the defendants fight tooth and nail over them because there are huge sums of money involved. For example, AstraZeneca paid $520 million for causing false claims by promoting Seroquel for use in children on Medicaid.

Psychiatrists and other MDs such as pediatricians who prescribe psychiatric drugs for reasons that are not medically indicated are guilty of Medicaid fraud because they *cause* the pharmacies to present (submit) false claims. These prescribing practices have been created by drug companies' relentless marketing of ineffective drugs for use with children and youth as depicted in Figure 6.1.

The government has pursued and obtained billions of dollars in False Claims Act and related criminal penalties from the drug companies at Step 1 of the Fraudulent Scheme but has thus far failed to pursue the psychiatrists at Step 2 or the pharmacies at Step 3. The problem with just going after the drug companies is that it doesn't stop psychiatrists and other prescribers from continuing to prescribe the drugs. In other words, the drug companies still rake in their profits from drugging poverty-stricken children and youth at government expense. The practical result from the settlements is that the drug companies cap their liability for the Medicaid fraud involved, meaning they won't have to pay any more. A recent study looking at the problem of illegal off-label promotion concluded "no regulatory strategy will be complete and effective without physicians themselves serving as a bulwark against off-label promotion."[31]

It is apparent that if the drug companies are causing false claims at Step 1, the psychiatrists are also causing false claims at Step 2, and the pharmacies are submitting false claims at Step 3. Any psychiatrist or other prescriber who regularly prescribes off-label psychotropic drugs to children and youth on Medicaid is likely to have written at least 1,000 prescriptions within the six-year statute of limitations, which would result in a judgment (order to pay) of $5.5 million.

Fraudulent Scheme

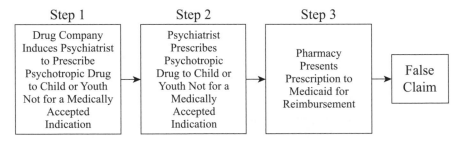

FIGURE 6.1.

In the belief that psychiatrists and other prescribers would quit the harmful practice of prescribing such psychotropic drugs to children and youth if they became aware that they face financial ruin for doing so, PsychRights launched an initiative to promote such lawsuits around the country in the summer of 2009. We developed a form that we call the "Model Complaint" designed for former foster youth to be the plaintiff (*relator*, technically) because so many of them have been victims of wrongful drugging.[32] However, anyone with information about specific offending prescriptions, such as parents, case workers, psychologists, teachers, counselors, and so forth, can use the Model Complaint form to support their efforts as a plaintiff (relator) in such a lawsuit. A list of which neuroleptics are approved for use with children, at what age, and for which diagnostic categories can be found on the Psychrights website. If a parent, psychologist, social worker, or any other caregiver knows of a child or youth on Medicaid who is being treated with a neuroleptic that is not listed, or is too young, or is being treated for a diagnosis for which the medication is not approved or supported by one of the compendia, it is Medicaid fraud, and they can become a plaintiff. In PsychRights' view, if a child or youth is given more than one psychiatric drug at a time, in what is called *polypharmacy*, it is also Medicaid fraud in almost all cases, regardless of the diagnosis or diagnoses.

— While psychiatrists and other prescribers tend not to have deep pockets, a tremendous amount of money could be won from the larger pharmacies. Pharmacies are therefore also included as defendants in the Model Complaint in order to attract attorneys to take these cases. The relator's share is between 15 and 30 percent of the recovery. People who might be in a position to bring such cases and attorneys interested in pursuing them are encouraged to contact PsychRights. Contact information is available at http://psychrights.org.

PsychRights has brought two such Medicaid fraud cases in Alaska,[33] and attorney Randy Kretchmar brought one in Illinois.[34] False Claims Act cases are initially sealed in order to allow the government time to investigate and decide whether to intervene and take over the case, and I anticipate more of such cases in the near future.[35]

The federal district court dismissed the Alaska cases on the grounds that the broad outline of the industry-wide fraud had been publicly disclosed, stating: the government already "has pursued False Claims Act cases and achieved extremely large recoveries against drug companies for causing the presentment of claims to Medicaid for prescriptions of psychotropic drugs that are not for medically accepted indications, including Geodon and Seroquel for use in children and youth."[36]

In other words, the federal district court dismissed the case because the government knows all about the fraud by psychiatrists and pharmacies. However, the government has not yet been compelled to do anything about it. PsychRights believes this decision is contrary to precedent, and the case has been appealed to the Ninth Circuit Court of Appeals, where briefing has been completed as of this writing in July 2011.[37] It is possible, but not likely, that the Ninth Circuit could decide the case within a few months. It will more likely take about a year.

In an unusual move, the Department of Justice moved to dismiss the *Nicholson* case in Illinois on the grounds that there were only five prescriptions involved and the case would not be worth the bother. This was proved to be untrue, but the court dismissed the case because the particular defendants apparently didn't have enough money to make it worthwhile. The court failed to consider certain things, such as the deterrence impact of such a case, but it is unknown at this time if the decision will be appealed.

HOW PARENTS AND MENTAL HEALTH PROFESSIONALS CAN PARTICIPATE IN LEGAL EFFORTS

Many parents and mental health professionals would like to participate in legal actions against the harmful use of neuroleptics and other psychiatric medications on children but don't know where or how to begin. Of critical importance is finding attorneys who are willing to take such cases. PsychRights is dedicated to taking on such cases, but its resources are limited. Every lawyer has an obligation to provide a certain amount of time *pro bono publico,* meaning volunteering legal services for people who cannot afford it. Most firms have pro bono programs that could be approached.

The Model Complaint for Medicaid fraud and the amount of money potentially available for attorneys make that an attractive approach. The key to such a case is that one has to have information about specific prescriptions submitted to Medicaid that were not for a medically accepted indication. Most prescriptions for neuroleptics to children and youth constitute Medicaid fraud. It is required that these cases be filed by attorneys.

State or § 1983 cases could be brought in states other than Alaska. Recruiting lawyers for such cases is important. §1983 does provide for an award of attorney's fees if one is successful, and there are lawyers who take §1983 cases.

There are also organizations of lawyers dedicated to protecting people's rights. The most well-known is the American Civil Liberties Union (ACLU). Historically, the ACLU has not been very supportive of adults trying to protect themselves from forced drugging, but protecting children is inherently more appealing, and it is worthwhile to approach your local ACLU for help. Other lawyer organizations devoted to protecting people's rights are the National Lawyers Guild and Lawyers for Public Justice. Protecting parents' right to make decisions regarding their children is one of the issues that the Rutherford Institute undertakes, and the Children's Defense Fund addresses children's issues as well.

In addition, each state has a federally funded agency "to protect and advocate for the rights of individuals with mental illness."[38] These protection and advocacy agencies (P&As) have special powers to investigate abuse and neglect of individuals diagnosed with mental illness and pursue administrative, legal, and other remedies. P&As have special standing rights. The P&As are a mixed bag, however, and often don't challenge the system.

The key to recruiting lawyers and organizations is to frame the request as a very important and beneficial thing to do. PsychRights has developed a memorandum aimed at recruiting such lawyers, which is available on its website (http://PsychRights.org).

If parents are saddled with public defenders who are not adequately representing their interests and those of their children, they can file a complaint with the local bar association. These lawyers are violating their ethical obligation to zealously represent the interests of their clients. Even on an individual basis, filing such complaints may help to get the type of representation people deserve. PsychRights stands ready to help people file such complaints because it may lend credibility to the complaint.

CONCLUSION

The horrific use of neuroleptics on defenseless children and youth cries out for legal efforts to curtail the practice. I have described the broad outlines of rights that children and youth have to be protected from harm and legal approaches to address the problem. The Medicaid fraud approach is like getting Al Capone for tax evasion, and we at PsychRights believe it has the potential to be extremely effective. The first cases are just now working their way through the courts, and if successful, it is expected that it will become relatively easy to recruit lawyers to take such cases. It is also important to recruit attorneys to take the other types of cases involving the wrongful use of psychiatric drugs on our youngest and most vulnerable citizens. The stakes are so high that anyone who cares about children and youth must do everything they can to protect them from this harm.

PART III

Drugging Our Children: Solutions

7

Drug-Free Mental Health Care for Children and Youth: Lessons from Residential Treatment

Tony Stanton

Eddie was sitting opposite his new teacher, Julie, when I walked into her class. This was my first chance to observe him as he had very recently entered our residential program. At age 7 he was a handsome little boy, on the skinny side, with unruly spiked blond hair. He initially seemed confused by this young lady who was paying such rapt attention to him. She had turned two of the student desks around so that they faced each other. Sitting in this little desk, she was as close as she could get to being on his level. Staff members were already going in and out of the classroom, and Eddie had no reason to pay attention to me—in any case, he was transfixed on Julie's face. As time went on, he was entranced. My guess is that he had never encountered anyone like this before. She was giving him her total quiet attention, asking about his past experiences in school and wondering what he really liked and didn't. Eddie, who was described in his referral as an "out of control and hyperactive" child, looked more like a little flower who had not been watered for a very long time. Over the next 45 minutes, he started to bloom; his expressions became livelier, and he began to smile as he answered her questions. A short time later, when he had rejoined the rest of the class, I heard him say to one of the other staff: "That's *my* teacher" with all the possessiveness he could muster. When I visited the classroom on later occasions I heard him, more than once, make the same comment: "That's *my* teacher"—pointing strongly, with his index finger, to Julie.

By the time Eddie entered our center, he had been taking antidepressant and antipsychotic medications for some time in the hope and belief that they would control his behaviors. As happened with most of the children referred to us, each increase in dose might slow them down for a couple of weeks, but they would inevitably return to their original behaviors. Also, typical of our referrals, there had been a reluctance to face the circumstances that had led to the symptoms in the first place: Eddie's hair-trigger defiance of adults. Beginning in infancy, more than 18 CPS reports had been filed on the family, and these had detailed serious physical and sexual abuse. Neither of his parents had received any help in their own lives—lives that had been torn by repeated abandonment, abuse, and eventual dependence on drugs and violence. Eddie had 10 placements before coming to our center. These included foster homes, group homes, and hospitalizations.

Certainly, Julie did not by herself perform a miraculous transformation; she had a sizable well-trained team backing her up. She did, however, utilize some of the more powerful ingredients that proved effective in the residential program: engaging a child in a real relationship, setting clear limits, and focusing on success in the present moment. For some time, Eddie was quick to get into struggles with staff. However, if this began to occur in class, Julie would calmly say his name or simply catch his eye. As soon as he noticed she was paying attention, little more was needed. He would look at her, stop whatever oppositional behavior he was engaged in, and return to the task at hand.

THE EXPERIMENT

Almost 24 years ago, I was asked to interview for a position as a child psychiatrist for a new subacute residence at an agency called Seneca Center, which served children in the Bay Area. The term *subacute* meant a residence that could treat the highest-need children— one step below a hospital. The CEO of the agency was behind this concept, and the psychologist assigned to the project had previously treated similar children. They were both alarmed that the treatment of so many children with behavioral symptoms was overly reliant on the use of psychiatric medication. It was their observation that these children responded well to a structured, safe environment with staff available to engage them. However, they were having difficulty finding a psychiatrist who would support a program that didn't resort to medication. I had previously directed a psychiatric unit in a hospital for several years. That program had been dedicated to the same principles treating much the same population. I was happy to participate in this new experiment.

When I was asked to write a chapter about our experiences in this program, children like Eddie and caregivers like Julie came to mind. Nevertheless, I had some skepticism: it was unclear to me whether my two and a half decades of work in a residential program would shed light on the current practice of using antipsychotic medications to treat an ever-expanding range of symptoms in even very young children. The population we treated was focused on the most behaviorally disordered children. Upon further reflection, however, I began to see that our experience does contribute an essential piece to the larger puzzle. In fact, the children we treated afford a particularly vivid understanding of the decisions that lead to the use of antipsychotic medication (and to the use of all categories of psychotropic medication). We treated more than 450 children over the past 24 years. Each one of them seriously challenged every attempt to help them. In a majority of cases, they had cycled through multiple failed placements, and psychiatric medication was the frontline intervention to address their aggression and unsafe behavior. Many clinicians would consider it a criminal act to deny such children psychotropic medication, and in a majority of cases, increasingly aggressive attempts had been made to suppress their symptoms with it. Some of our children had undergone trials with as many 18 different medications. Most were still being prescribed 4 or 5 when admitted to our care.

We offered both short-and long-term stays—some as short as two to three months or as long as four years. Our bottom-line experience was that even the most seriously disturbed children responded to the high level of care we provided. This was possible because our program had the capacity to engage their behaviors while highlighting their capacities for success. In contrast, the facilities that referred the children to us did not have the staffing, structure, or philosophy to intervene effectively. Lacking these essential ingredients, these programs became heavily dependent on medication—particularly for those children that posed the greatest challenges.

One important consequence of having such high-quality staff resources was our ability to give children a message they had never heard before, a message that became a key ingredient of success. This message was not announced to the child. It was an *action*, not a *saying*. However, if asked to put it into words, we could express it as follows:

"In the past you have had many placements because the people caring for you found your behavior intolerable and they did not feel capable of intervening meaningfully. You will never be discharged from our program for this reason. You have been told that there is something wrong with your brain and that this prevents you from being in control of your own actions. We don't believe that. We are gradually going to remove these medications because we believe you have the capacity for success and that you can learn to be in charge of your own actions."

One of the first things most children did when they entered our program was to test us and see if we could keep them. They would throw their worst behavior at us to find out if we could deal with it. When I first saw Denzel, age 7, with his therapist, Susan, we had said little more than "hello" when he rushed at me and attacked me in every way he knew how: punching, kicking, spitting. I held him for more than 30 minutes so that he could not hurt me until he calmed down. My experience with Denzel was one of many of his tests—after a couple of weeks he realized that he was not going to be discharged, and he began making trusting relationships with staff whom, at first, he labeled as "mean."

Establishing a New Paradigm of Evaluation

Shortly after we initiated our program, we started evaluating children using an approach that was in sharp contrast to most of our colleagues. We began to amass every bit of history we could find, both from records and from interviews. We then assembled this into a chronological table that displayed a summary of this information in linear sequence. We did this before writing an evaluation.

Most of the records we reviewed were like snapshots. There were, on average, 30 such documents for each child (amounting to more than 13,000 documents for 450 children seen in the course of 23 years). Almost all of these documents (psychological evaluations, CPS reports, court reports, hospital evaluations, to name a few) ended up as isolated pictures of some particular aspect of the child's life. The task for me was to discover the narrative behind these reports and to string together the snapshots so that they finally began to resemble something more like a movie—a movie that, up until then, had been hidden. This led us to become detectives who sought out what was missing in these children's life histories. It became clear through time that what was of lesser importance in a child's past had been displayed prominently, while what was of greatest importance was, more often than not, left out.

We found that the narratives with greatest explanatory power, the ones needing to be displayed most prominently, were those describing the elements of safety and quality of relationships in the earliest years of the child's life. Researchers in child development, over the past 50 years, have been exhaustively studying these elements (see "Putting Real Science to Work" below). Their findings confirmed our own: the factors that determine children's capacity to form relation-ships and regulate their own lives are found in the histories of their earliest relationships.

This contrasts with much of the current wisdom guiding the treat-ment of disturbed children. This wisdom favors a belief that the main determinants of their difficulties reside in biological brain disorders and that these, in turn, have significant genetic determinants. These were the assumptions that guided the treatment of the children re-ferred to us. They remain the default assumptions in our culture.

Mark: A Case Example

One of our first clients offers an excellent illustration of these as-sumptions. At the time of his referral, he was nine years old, taking a standard antipsychotic at a dose 10 times the usual initial amount rec-ommended for a psychotic adult. This was given, ostensibly, to treat a psychosis. However, neither his history nor our observations revealed evidence of a psychosis. Early on, we noticed that he took little care of his appearance and tried to avoid engaging adults and peers alike. His history showed that he had difficulties in preschool and would strike out at peers and he had difficulty following routines. We began to no-tice that any loud noise or an unexpected fall would result in intense fear reactions. Once he experienced this fear, he could not tolerate comfort from adults. As he stated to one of his teachers, "I don't like to be near people when I get hurt": He evidently believed that caretakers would make things worse. This pattern remained unchanged by the antipsychotic medication.

Prior to his referral to us, he had a succession of increasingly re-strictive placements—in hospitals and residential settings. He became more and more threatening to his peers and parents. With every place-ment failure, he was prescribed higher doses of medication. In each instance, it was concluded that his acting out was due to a psychotic process treated with inadequate doses of antipsychotic medication. When it became clear to the funding agencies that they would have to pay more for hospitalizations than for our residence, he was placed in our care.

This was a frequent theme in our children's histories: the failure to note that the medications were simply not working. Various symp-toms were interpreted as proof that a child suffered from psychosis. Very often these could be voices that the child heard or, as in this case, a preoccupation with fantasy figures. Medication then became a medi-cal necessity. When Mark first came to us he was very slow and had little spontaneity. We also confirmed his most striking behavior: He would start to get upset, perhaps start to throw things, at which point staff would begin to calmly get closer to him. He would then say, "Stay away from me." This pattern repeated itself over and over.

We knew that Mark's mother had been under severe stress at the time of Mark's birth and during his first years of life. We did not know, however, that there was a more precise origin of his fear—a fear of physical intimacy that was most pronounced when he was in a state of anxiety. Then, quite by accident, we learned a critical clue. We did not need this detail to treat Mark. However, in putting together the picture puzzle of his life, we were given this missing piece that allowed us to see a much more complete picture of his earlier life.

It happened in this way: One of us participated in a meeting about another child with a therapist in the community. This therapist heard that Mark had been transferred into our program. He had tried to help Mark and his mother when Mark was still an infant. At that time, Mark's mother had described extremely disturbing interactions with her son, interactions that were repeated over and over again. Mark would get upset and begin crying. Mother would find that she could not calm him down, and the crying would escalate. Finally mother would grab him and scream at him as loud as she could. At that point Mark would freeze and just stop moving or crying. The therapist regretted that he had only been able to work with this family for a very short period of time and had lost track of them. Although Mark's father had been in the home, he was incapable of emotionally supporting Mark's mother, nor was there any available support from the extended family.

We could not have found a clearer corollary between Mark's behaviors and this early developmental trauma—in this case, a series of specific traumas that took place between him and his mother. This was not a trauma that was going to be cured with psychotropic medication.

Ingredients for Success

As noted above, children referred to us on psychotropic medications had been treated primarily for disorganized or aggressive behavior. On occasion, as in the case of Mark, they were diagnosed with symptoms of psychosis. In essence, medications had been used in settings that did not have the essential ingredients for effective treatment. This certainly was the case with Mark. Soon after he entered our, care he began to defy staff and demand that they stay away from him. At the same time, he seemed relieved when they led him, with little more than a touch on his shoulders, to a quieter place where he calmed down. This sequence was repeated many times and slowly; he gained more and more control of himself. The reductions in his medications had the reverse effect of his parents' fears. He became more available, more alert, and more engaged with staff. He also noticed that we had a larger interest in who he was beyond his symptoms—he noticed that we appreciated his interests, talents, and intelligence. His parents, however, remained extremely fearful that the reductions in medication would make it impossible for him to live with them if he returned home.

Described below are the essential ingredients utilized in the residential program. Children who exhibit disorganized and aggressive behavior require high levels of regulation and consistency. To achieve these, we needed a high staff/child ratio and staff who were well trained. It was also important to maintain close collaboration with parents, courts, and any social agencies that had legal custody of the child. These staffing and collaborative ingredients were necessary both in the residence and in our school.

One of the most important ingredients in successful residential treatment is ordinarily not described as an ingredient at all: the process of evaluation. As stated above, what ordinarily passes for an evaluation is a history of symptoms combined with a cursory and imprecise history of relationships. While this is in part due to financial constraints dictating less and less time for evaluation, it has also become the standard of care.

By carefully assembling histories and following up clues, as we did with Mark, we were able to identify the types of engagement that were going to be most helpful. We know from our experience (and from the literature on child development that has burgeoned over the last 40 years) that a child's capacity to regulate himself, to feel secure, and to explore the world are critically dependent on the quality of his relationships in the earliest years. If a family is mired in abuse, chaos, or neglect, and they have no help or support, the children are seriously impacted.

Jane, who entered our program at age 10, had been sexually assaulted by her mother's boyfriend. This fact had been played down and hidden in the reports. Mother was determined to have Jane returned to her as soon as possible but kept giving her daughter (and us) veiled clues that her boyfriend was still involved. Jane heard her mother make a passing comment about this and put together other clues indicating he was still around. We noted that Jane was becoming increasingly upset after any contact with her mother. Finally, this untenable situation was acknowledged by the social agencies in charge of her placement. They made it clear to Jane that they would never return her to such an unsafe environment. It was at this point that she began to make greater progress in the program. When Jane was referred to us, she was on three medications: a stimulant, an antidepressant, and an antipsychotic. Previous evaluations had focused on a theory that Jane had brain damage while ignoring the issue of safety.

Ray came to us at age 11 after "blowing out" of all previous programs attempting to treat him. His evaluations stressed, over and over, that his behaviors were due to bipolar disorder. When we carefully reviewed the previous evaluations, we found one written by a psychologist who had seen the family when Ray was not yet 5. He focused on the interactions between Ray and his parents. He noted that the parents were not abusive but that they had totally failed to set any limits on his behavior. Thus, at an early age, he became a tyrant in his own family. Our assessment confirmed the findings of the earlier psychologist and made it clear that he was neither an abused child nor did he have a brain disorder. He soon learned that he could not control our staff. As time went on he and the staff discovered that he was an exceedingly bright and engaging child who had basically been embalmed with medication by the time of his admission—at that point, he was taking five medications including two mood stabilizers, an antidepressant, an antipsychotic, and a stimulant. Later, after his parents had done a great deal of work in learning new ways of setting limits, he was able to return home.

THE RESULTS: OUTCOMES

An inevitable question gets posed (in particular by those who are impressed by statistical results): what percentage of children improved in our program and what were their outcomes after they left our program? The statistics are simple. First, all the children referred to us experienced failure in their previous placements. Second, they all improved while in our care. No child was ever discharged from our care because of their disruptive behaviors.

How did we measure this success? In the case of each child, we have meticulous records of their behavior in the residence and school, their relationships with peers and staff, and their relationships to their families. We can point out what worked and how we learned from what didn't—notably, medication. Colleagues will often say, "OK, they improved in your care, but what happened afterward?" Understandably, they want *outcome studies*. What was their rate of success in subsequent placements? That success varied a great deal. The key ingredient was the wisdom of those in charge of the subsequent placements. In some cases, children were returned to settings that were clearly unsafe, and many of their behaviors returned—behaviors that were their best efforts to protect themselves.

The question regarding outcomes, however, contains an assumption that is endemic to the current treatment culture. It is the assumption that we can fix children with some specific intervention, which will then immunize them from any further difficulties. Most outcome studies are focused on specific symptoms, not quality of life.

Several myths about our program were heard over the years. One was that we succeeded by simply having a strict behavioral system. Another asserted that we simply overwhelmed children with large staff who could physically restrain them. We did utilize a behavioral system, and we did utilize staff members who were trained and capable of managing any aggressive behavior that the children might manifest. Children definitely responded to staff when they experienced them as people who could safely contain them. If this containment required them to be held, they would learn over time that this holding was not a form of retaliation or abuse (which they had often experienced in the past) but an engagement that was carried out solely for the purpose of helping them regain a sense of safety and regulation within themselves.

Although I didn't prescribe psychotropic medication for these children, there were many requests for them. I personally took requests for medication very seriously as, ironically, they often led to more effective interventions. A request for medication could arise from our own staff, from parents, and from social agencies. Once we could describe which behaviors we were being asked to medicate, we could become more curious about the origin and settings where these behaviors were seen. Questions such as the following were pursued: Were there settings where the behaviors were not in evidence? Did the behaviors diminish when the child was with certain staff? Had there been critical changes in staff, peers, the school, family visits, or discharge plans? At times, I would also consult colleagues and ask if they had any ideas about specific medications that would help in this specific situation. Each request for medication led to a new evaluation of the child. We were always able to identify the elements missing in the child's treatment. When we provided these elements, the child responded and the request for medication was dropped.

While the program utilized structure and predictable patterns of engagement with all the children, it would be a serious error to believe that we were able to just plug children into the program and fix them. Each child we saw forced us to develop a new treatment to address his or her unique challenges. What was common to all success, however, was the child forming trusting relationships with particular staff. For many, this was their first experience of being seen, treasured, and held in the mind of an adult.

LESSONS FROM OUR "NEUROBIOLOGICAL CULTURE"

When we established our program, we worked toward creating clearer pictures of children's actual lives. This included the circumstances and relationships that they experienced each year of their lives as well as histories of their parents. In the process, another picture began to emerge: a picture of the culture that these parents and children lived in. We had not planned on creating this picture. It happened as an accident, a by-product of gathering as much information as possible on each child. Thousands of documents, with very few exceptions, revealed agencies sharing the same conceptual deficits in the assumptions and theories they applied to the children they treated, tried to protect, or placed. A description of these conceptual deficits, however, was not found in the documents. They remained unstated, in the background, as they have become endemic to the larger culture. These *conceptual deficits* include the following: the neglect of curiosity, the fear of blame, the demise of empathic imagination, and attribution of identity through diagnosis.

When these deficits are made explicit, they reveal approaches to protection, diagnosis, and treatment of children that promote less and less engagement and curiosity. The bottom line becomes "identify the symptoms, find the diagnosis, and treat with the indicated psychiatric medication."

Just as individuals can be unconscious of their motives in carrying out certain actions in their lives, our society as a whole wears a set of blinders when it comes to the reality of children's lives—including those children referred to us for the highest level of care. Our society has also become blind to the poor efficacy of the biological treatments that are now considered the state-of-the-art treatments. This has been documented in great detail in Robert Whitaker's book *Anatomy of an Epidemic*.[1] The epidemic he describes reminds me of the "collective disease" affecting the population in the Hans Christian Anderson fairy tale: they were told, and came to believe, that the emperor was wearing increasingly refined clothes when, in fact, he was wearing none at all.

What follows is a description of the assumptions in the culture enumerated above.

The Death of Curiosity

Some years ago, staff requested that I do training on psychotropic medication. My colleague and I concluded that it would be far more useful to do a training on *curiosity*. He did the major work in constructing this training, which described ways to foster curiosity when so many elements in our current therapeutic climate conspire to destroy it. Most of the subjects described in this chapter were covered in that training.

One of the first things we observed in the records sent to us was a death of curiosity. This was due, in part, to the rush to impose a diagnostic label. Once the diagnosis was applied, curiosity was no longer necessary. The goal had been reached: the child's behaviors and symptoms were placed in their proper category. In the records sent to us, we saw the repeated implication that there was nothing left to describe or discover. In particular, the child's living connections with caretakers and their history had become irrelevant. A logical result was that clues about the origins of symptoms, like those we found for Mark or Jim, didn't need to be pursued.

Some of the most tragic results of such assessments involved attempts to treat children in settings that were manifestly unsafe for the child. Sometimes this took place in a home where the interventionist failed to realize that the child was regularly or intermittently placed in contact with a person who was actively abusing her. In other cases, the evaluation failed to determine that the parent who had custody never had a secure relationship with the child in the first place.

Once a child failed to improve, she was given a more serious diagnosis such as bipolar disorder or psychosis NOS (not otherwise specified) reflecting escalating and recalcitrant behavior. This paved the way for more potent psychiatric medication—including mood stabilizers and antipsychotics. This pattern is exemplified by a child I saw in a community mental health agency. He had been raised in his earliest years of life by his mother, in a highly abusive environment, and had to be removed from her care. Later, he was returned to her care on the basis that she had reformed. The treatment team, however, failed to be curious about the distressed nature of the original bond between the boy and his mother. His early experiences of insecurity with her had been embedded in his nervous system, and there was no way that she could offer him the security he needed. This led to higher and higher levels of medication. With each new medication, or increase in dose, he was temporarily slowed down, but with time, all proved ineffective. Eventually, he had to be removed from her care permanently. By that time, both he and his mother had been highly traumatized by their inability to make things work.

As noted above, children who came into our residential care did not automatically improve. Often, there was persistent aggression or dangerous behavior such as running away. These were all opportunities to look more closely. We held special meetings, looked more carefully at every aspect of the child's life, and did not cease in this endeavor until we had, in fact, discovered which factors needed to be addressed. John, age 10, seemed to be relentlessly aggressive. At first, we had erratic success in addressing it. We finally honed in on the fact that one particular staff member had, indeed, great success in engaging this boy. This allowed other staff to identify the ingredients of success in this relationship. We also noted that he was much more aggressive after visits with his mother. Although she was in no position to reunify with him, it became clear that she was giving him the message that he would soon return to her care. He began to experience greater success in our program when this issue was addressed.

Blame and the Demise of Empathic Imagination

A major factor governing current evaluations of children's difficulties is the fear of blaming parents. Agencies will go to great lengths to avoid any inference that would indicate that parents have a connection to their children's disturbances. The increasing assertion that children's difficulties are primarily due to biological and genetic conditions means that parents can be assured that their own lives and their interactions with their children play no role. The most destructive result of this paradigm is that it leads parents to believe that they have no agency with their own children. As a result, most of the families referred to us had been given little to no help. Many of them had been subject to an unrelenting series of traumas but few interventions that went beyond threats of removing their children. Most of these parents had suffered serious abuse and neglect in their own backgrounds, and high percentages were subject to substance abuse, poverty, and serial abusive relationships. Avoiding blame and asserting a purely biological paradigm, deprived them of learning how to engage their child's behavior. Biological certainty had replaced opportunity. They didn't get help when it would have helped most: early on.

The solution to this dilemma was expressed in a quote from Jeree Pawl:[2] "We learn over time that everything we think we know is a hypothesis; that we have ideas, but that we don't have truth . . . When we know this, our attitude conveys it; and the child and family sense themselves as sources, not objects. In this context, they become aware of a mutual effort. They do not feel weighed, measured or judged. They do feel listened to, seen and appreciated."

Fear of blame can not only destroy the possibility of creative engagement, but it can also lead to the demise of what I call *empathic imagination*: the capacity to imagine, through time and circumstances, the effect of destructive relationships on a child. While most people can summon up this imaginative capacity when someone describes experiences of being incarcerated and tortured in a prison camp, they can lose this ability with a child despite a clear history that the child was subject to long periods of neglect, abuse, or unpredictable environments in their first three years of life. Many professionals, particularly those held in thrall of the current biological models, seem to forget that lack of security in earliest development results in the most devastating neurological and psychological damage for the child.

Attributions of Identity

A frequent element seen in our referral records was the act of fixing a child's identity with a diagnosis. Curiosity about a child's unique personality and traits was replaced with a label. Ray, the child described above, was given a diagnosis after he was observed as being "out of control." When all pharmaceutical interventions had proved ineffective, he was referred to a department of child psychiatry in a prominent university. After evaluating him, they began their report by stating, "This 11-year-old boy with known bipolar disorder." Thus, his identity had been determined through his diagnosis, and this became the most important factor in knowing who he was.

Most children who came into our care had similar histories of losing their identities to a diagnosis. In some cases, they would end up describing themselves in these terms. Some were amazed if we questioned this. After all, many evaluations had affirmed the seriousness of their condition—they *were* that label. Some also seriously questioned our plan to remove the medications that were supposed to be treating their diagnosis. One girl, Trish, announced that if we dared to remove her medication, we would discover just how destructive she could be: she was bipolar; she would destroy our program. Three weeks later, her parents came for a visit. During the intervening time, her medication had been largely discontinued, and her aggression had been successfully engaged. We were getting to know her, and she was becoming freer in showing us who she was. As her parents entered the room, Trish announced to them: "These people know what they are doing."

PUTTING REAL SCIENCE TO WORK

If our larger culture has embraced a simplistic view of human development and has disregarded the impact of experience and relationship, is there an alternative view? The alternative is alive and quite vigorous. When I speak of an alternative science, or real science, I am referring to several bodies of professional literature that describe human lives, the development of persons, and the neurophysiology of development and emotion. It is also a literature that describes the circumstances that lead to disorganized lives and aggression.

Great efforts were put forth to make this information available to the residential staff who worked with our children. It is the antidote to all simplistic thinking that infects the wider culture's views of children's difficulties. This information is not readily found in the media. There, you are more likely to find an ad for the latest medication to cure your child's attention deficit/hyperactivity disorder (ADHD) or bipolar disorder. Although the real science has been rendered virtually invisible to the general public, it has quietly developed into a large body of knowledge. It also happens to verify what one of my teachers once described as "a grandmother's common sense."

In the 1950s, John Bowlby published his groundbreaking research on the subject of *attachment*, children's earliest relationships with their caregivers.[3] His work illuminated the central influence that the quality of the mother-child relationship has on all aspects of children's development, as a blueprint for future relationships, language development, as well as their capacity for creativity expressed through play, and their ability to learn. His research has been replicated, expanded upon, and refined over the past 60 years, and attachment research has become a cornerstone of the child development field.

One of the first clinicians to intervene in early parenting gone awry was Selma Fraiberg who chronicled her work in *Clinical Studies in Infant Mental Health*.[4] A more recent, comprehensive book describing such "parent-infant therapy" is *Psychotherapy with Infants and Young Children* by Alicia Lieberman and Patricia Van Horn.[5] Of interest is the fact that this book has no references to psychotropic medication at all. While the pharmaceutical industry targets younger and younger children, many therapists are finding that the principles of parent-infant therapy are powerful ingredients in the treatment of older children.

More recently, with the aid of brain imaging techniques, neuropsychological research has rendered the impact of attachment relationships on children's developing brains visible. This research demonstrates that infant-caregiver relationships are the single most powerful environmental influence on brain development in the early years. Through extensive and detailed neuropsychological research, Alan Schore affirmed the assertion made by the child psychiatrist Winnicott many decades ago: "There is no such thing as a baby—there is always a baby and mother."* The child's nervous system is sculpted through each interaction with its mother.[6] Writers and clinicians such as Daniel Siegal, Bruce Perry, and Daniel Stern have written a number of books describing the impact of the quality of care that infants receive on their developing brains for those who may not have extensive medical knowledge.[7] Nature has its place, but nurture turns out to be the critical ingredient when it comes to ensuring healthy brain development and a child's agency in the larger world.

A very different body of research leads us from the world of neurology into the common pathway of human interaction: the importance of the *stories of relationships*—making sense of what has happened and promoting more creative stories for the future. Robert Coles, in 1989, highlighted this theme most beautifully in a book called *The Call of Stories*.[8] He began the book by describing his training as a resident assigned to work with a "difficult patient," a patient who refused to talk to him. Some of his supervisors recommended that he focus on finding out which symptoms she suffered from. One supervisor, however, encouraged him to simply "listen to her story." When he offered simply to listen she became quite alive and transformed. Acknowledging the importance of the opportunity to "tell your story" and having someone listen to it respectfully is a critical ingredient for healing all disturbed children. It makes all the difference in residential treatment.

THE UNFINISHED COPERNICAN REVOLUTION[9]

For 14 centuries, the official scientific view held that the sun went around the earth. This was known as the Ptolemaic theory. Since actual observations indicated the opposite, increasingly complex mathematical equations were marshaled for support. By the time Copernicus challenged this theory, it had grown into an immense edifice of complexity. Given that it was also a bulwark of church doctrine (that God created the earth as the center of the universe), it could cost a person his life to challenge it. Copernicus avoided this fate by making sure his work was not published before his death.

Today, we are witnessing a similar resistance to explanations of human development and psychological difficulties in spite of the fact that they are based on rigorous research. The ascendant theory, advanced by a powerful industry, asserts that children and adults who

---

* The term *mother* refers to anyone who serves as a child's primary caregiver or *attachment* figure, whether it be the biological or adoptive mother, father, grandparent, and so forth.

exhibit problems in living are suffering from discreet disease states—basically identical to physical illnesses. Since these are defined as brain disorders, it is argued that the only effective treatment is medical. This view places the center of explanation within the child's brain: her neurophysiology and genetic heritage. Her difficulties are believed to be totally separate from her family history, school environment, and cultural influences. As a result, she is stripped of her story except for the one that might indicate the biological forces that have been at work, autonomously, within her genes and nervous system.

When I assert this as the ascendant paradigm, I am not suggesting that all therapists, including psychiatrists, are totally under its sway. There are strong traditions in every therapeutic discipline that affirm the importance of both history and relationship. There are many therapists who address the actual lives of their clients. These therapists and traditions, however, are increasingly drowned out in the arena of public discourse, by the current Ptolemaic view.

Ironically, the next Copernican revolution, when it does arrive, will highlight a much more authentic science, a science drawing upon the expansive literature alluded to above—describing all manner of correlations between the vicissitudes of human relationships, development, and neurophysiology. For the moment, however, this literature remains out of sight for those who could most benefit from its use. Given the tenacious forces promoting the current Ptolemaic theory, it is not clear when or how a Copernican theory of human development and conflict will assert itself, or when it will begin to marshal forces for a serious challenge to what is currently privileged as a bible of religious truth.

As more attention is paid to the real circumstances impacting families and children, earlier interventions will be utilized. When this happens, we will see far fewer children who need the intense levels of intervention described in this chapter.

THE CHALLENGE FACING PARENTS AND CARETAKERS

Currently, many sectors within the health system are relentlessly promoting biological models of mental illness as the cause of all difficulties in human living and, at the same time, offering psychiatric drugs as the primary cure. These sectors include the most powerful institutions in the medical establishment: those that train doctors, nurses, and psychiatrists, together with the pharmaceutical industry. Their biases are amplified by multimillion-dollar ad campaigns and stories in the media about the diagnosis du jour and the latest blockbuster drug. They are effectively drowning out less powerful voices that offer highly effective approaches to treating children's behavioral and emotional challenges. As a consequence, psychiatric medication as a first-line approach to treatment has become the norm. A majority of parents now assume that the biological model with its attendant medications is the last word in describing and treating their children's emotional difficulties because it is the only word they hear.

Nonetheless, many parents whose children have been prescribed psychiatric medication have arrived at their own conclusions about the limitations of drug-based therapies. They are unwilling to reduce their children's behaviors and feelings to so many misfired neurons, and they have witnessed firsthand the myriad side effects of their children's psychiatric drugs. They are seeking advice about whether it is safe to forgo psychiatric drugs altogether or to wean their children from drugs that they are already on. I have no simple formula to address these concerns. Formulaic thinking is in fact one of the key limitations of the biological approach. Just as each child in our care needed individual treatment approaches, all children in need of help from a mental health professional require interventions that are tailored to their unique circumstances and personalities. I can however, recommend that parents come armed with the following set of questions for the prescribing physician. Answers to these questions will help parents to make informed choices:

1. What are your beliefs about mental health and illness, and how do you understand the cause of my child's difficulties?
2. Are you prescribing medication to treat my child's symptoms or to treat a disease?
3. Are there specific changes that I can look for in my child's behavior that would indicate the medication is no longer needed?
4. Are you recommending psychotherapy along with medication? If so, what type and will we (the parents) be involved as well?

These questions will help parents to clearly establish which behaviors have contributed to the diagnostic label(s) that their child was assigned, and to consider whether these behaviors are indeed symptoms of a disease or their child's attempt to solve an actual dilemma in his or her life. The latter happened to be the case for all the children we treated in our residence.

The second question highlights a critical distinction. Historically, we have seen two major rationales for prescribing psychiatric medication to children. The first was to take the edge off, to help the child get through a difficult time. This was conceived as a time-limited intervention that would no longer be necessary when the child had learned to develop control over his or her own feelings and behavior. This rationale was expressed very clearly in a paper written by Melvin Lewis in 1978.[10] He described the process of making decisions about medication in a residential program he was running at the time: "A misunderstanding that was often encountered in staff discussions of whether to employ a drug was the notion that it was being used to control the child: In fact, the purpose of using a drug was to help the child control himself or herself." Careful observation will confirm that Dr. Lewis's intentions are rarely adhered to in the current culture. Control of the child rather than self-control is most often the purpose of such interventions. This is particularly true in school settings. The second, increasingly common rationale for giving a child psychotropic medication is to treat a medical disease. Diagnoses such as ADHD, bipolar disorder, autistic spectrum disorders, or psychosis (to name a few) are often presumed to be genetic brain diseases. Such assumptions render children candidates for lifelong medication.

As noted above, our experience was mainly with children who had serious behavioral disturbances. Almost all were given diagnoses such as ADHD, bipolar disorder, and psychoses—sometimes all three. Since these children were a good cross-section of the most out-of-control children in our state one would assume that some of them must have been prime examples of children with biological disorders. Yet even the most disturbed responded well to engagement with our staff. A standard joke in our program was that we cured all bipolar children sent to us. We ended up agreeing with the authors writing in Sharna Olfman's book *Bipolar Children* that this is a nefarious diagnosis.[11] Can children be psychotic? Indeed, they can be, but it is exceedingly rare. Most children now diagnosed as psychotic are given that designation because of symptoms such as hearing a voice, which, in our experience, was always related to dissociated experiences (someone's voice from the past). Psychotic symptoms inevitably disappeared as the children became engaged with staff.

When parents question the advisability of a psychiatric drug that their child is already using, it is neither easy nor expedient to immediately take charge from the physician and abruptly wean the child from the medication. First, this could lead to serious withdrawal effects, and second, parents need to be sure that an effective alternative treatment plan is in place. Effective treatment always includes a focus on facilitating healthy relationships and establishing supportive settings. This is possible to initiate whether or not a child has been placed on medication. Although parents have the right to request that their child terminate use of psychiatric medication, they will feel more secure in making a collaborative plan with the physician when they can share information indicating that the symptoms targeted by the medication can be engaged and changed.

It is my hope that in the near future parents will have liberal access to sound information about children's mental health. This will encourage them to seek out professionals who do not rely heavily on psychiatric medication so that they are not saddled with the complexities of then weaning their child from unnecessary and potentially harmful drugs. I recommend that parents look for professionals in their community who will conduct a thorough evaluation of their child's difficulties. A comprehensive evaluation will attempt to identify the settings and relationships that have contributed to their child's distress, as well as relationships and environments that will enable their child to experience success without medications. If, for example, a teacher complains about a child's disruptive behavior in the classroom and urges the parents to seek help, instead of working with a pediatrician or psychiatrist who is quick to pull out the prescription pad, they can instead look for a mental health professional who will evaluate the extent to which the teacher, classmates, and family members as well as the wider school and home environment may be contributing to the problem, in addition to identifying the people with whom, and the settings in which, the child is thriving. It is also important to seek out a mental health professional who will engage parents as partners—who can help them find clues to their children's difficulties, clues that will help them and their children to meaningfully engage those difficulties.

FINAL THOUGHTS

As I noted earlier, the residential program described in this chapter is a program within an agency known as Seneca Center. Under the exceptional leadership of its CEO, Ken Berrick, the agency has expanded into a wide variety of programs for children and their families with an increasing focus on early intervention. The agency has remained committed to a philosophy of care favoring community, school, and family engagement over psychotropic medication. The two gentlemen—Ken Berrick and John Sprinson—who originally hired me have written a book describing many elements of the treatment model utilized in the agency.[12]

Unfortunately, the residential program is heavily dependent on funding from the state and counties of California, and the budgets of these governmental agencies have diminished significantly over the years. As a result, this program has been steadily forced to cut services and currently cares for only a few children. With the ongoing budgetary crisis in California, it may eventually have to close. Children not served by our program will, more likely than not, be forced into care where there will be less structure and more medication.

It is time for all mental health professionals who are alarmed by the excessive use of psychiatric medication with children to find the courage and commitment to take action against this dangerous trend and to make their values and knowledge more accessible so that parents can find effective and safe interventions for their children without first wading through the often treacherous waters of psychiatric drugs. Indeed, all of us who care about children need to work toward a paradigm shift within the mental health system—one that engages children's lives and supports humane and effective care.

8

Strategic Family Therapy as an Alternative to Antipsychotics

George Stone

It is hard work to see what is in front of your nose.

—George Orwell

There has been a 1,000-fold increase in the number of American children labeled mentally ill since the first antipsychotic drugs were introduced in the 1950s. At that time, only 7,500 children were diagnosed as psychiatrically disturbed, and the newly minted antipsychotics were targeted to adult schizophrenics. Today, more than 8 million children have a psychiatric diagnosis, and antipsychotics have become a blockbuster drug for the treatment of a host of children's behavioral issues. By 2008, antipsychotic drugs topped sales in all other categories because of skyrocketing prescriptions to children in spite of the fact that they are known to reduce quality of life and shorten life span. Furthermore, psychotherapy has been shown to be as effective for treating psychiatric disturbance as drugs in the short term and *more* effective in the long term.[1] One measure of a society's values is how it treats its most vulnerable members. The indiscriminate marketing of dangerous drugs for use with children in order to shore up the bottom line speaks to the primacy of corporate greed in American society.

THE MEDICALIZATION OF CHILDHOOD

In 1976, the late Henry Gadsden, then CEO of Merck Pharmaceuticals, gave a candid interview to *Fortune* magazine. Frustrated that his company's potential markets were "limited to sick people," he dreamed that Merck would one day become like Wrigley's chewing gum and "sell to everyone." Today, Gadsden's dream has been realized; drug makers are indeed "selling to everyone," including American children.[2]

Aided and abetted by America's legendary faith in medical progress and by new regulations that weakened corporate oversight, in the 1980s the pharmaceutical industry began to aggressively target healthy people in all sectors of American society including children. By reframing or medicalizing undesirable behaviors and moods as illness and disorder and marketing these new diagnoses to the American public, drug manufacturers were then able to significantly increase sales of a burgeoning number of drugs that were alleged to confer health and happiness on its users. Children's naturally shifting moods and limited attention spans were pathologized as a vehicle for drug sales. The pharmaceutical industry hit upon a winning formula: selling sickness sells drugs.[3]

Drug companies accomplish their goal of "selling to everyone" by stacking the scientific deck in their favor. The pharmaceutical industry funds its own research and heavily subsidizes medical training and medical literature. It also salaries a significant numbers of employees in the FDA—the very agency designed to police the industry. Its reach even extends to the *Diagnostic and Statistical Manual* (*DSM-IV TR*), commonly referred to as the bible of psychiatry because an overwhelming majority of mental health practitioners rely on it as their primary source for diagnostic guidelines.[4] The *DSM* is not the scientific treatise that it is purported to be, but rather a political document that publishes psychiatric diagnoses that are defined by consensus among panels of psychiatrists, the majority of whom are consultants to drug companies. The pharmaceutical industry rigs consensus by offering panel members stock options, speaker's fees, and research grants. In return, panelists need only agree to include a new diagnostic category, or to expand the boundaries of an existing disorder. At the same time, consensus can be swayed to restrict "best practice" recommendations to treatment protocols that favor drug therapies over psychotherapies.[5] In chapter 4, former pharmaceutical industry insider Gwen Olsen provides a vivid description of how drug makers design and fund research that supports new disorders, and markets them alongside the drugs allegedly designed to treat them. And in chapter 1, Robert Whitaker furnishes a chilling case example of how thought leaders in psychiatry, heavily funded by the pharmaceutical industry, created the pediatric bipolar disorder epidemic that catalyzed record-breaking sales of antipsychotics for use with children.

In addition to the obvious harm done when children are wrongly diagnosed and prescribed dangerous drugs, a more subtle but equally damaging process is at work. When children's emotional turmoil or problematic behaviors are medicalized, their caregivers are encouraged to believe that psychiatric drugs are all that is needed to treat their children's illnesses. A concomitant set of beliefs is that psychotherapy is unnecessary and parents do not have a meaningful role to play in helping their children with their behavioral and emotional challenges, aside from ensuring compliance with the drug regimen. Recent research demonstrated that parents whose children were given a prescription for a stimulant drug and then told to enroll their child in an attention-deficit/hyperactivity disorder (ADHD) behavioral intervention program actually did so only 25 percent of the time. In contrast, parents told by their doctor to enroll their child in an ADHD behavioral intervention program *before* using drugs did so 95 percent of the time. In a separate study, Medco Health Solutions tracked 5,000 children for three months following an initial prescription of an antidepressant and found that more than 50 percent of these children had not had a single psychotherapy session.[6]

Alchemy is an ancient tradition whose practitioners were on a quest for a fabled elixir that was capable of turning base metals into gold and maintaining eternal youth. Alchemy is also an allegory for the spiritual quest for ultimate wisdom.[7] It appears that the alchemist's dream of an elixir that creates gold was realized—for the pharmaceutical industry in any event—by medicalizing human suffering. However, medicalization has turned the alchemists' companion dreams of eternal youth and ultimate wisdom into nightmares. Today's elixirs are significantly reducing life expectancy and narrowing our vision of the human condition to the physiological events occurring inside the human body to the exclusion of the rich and complex human relationships that give life meaning and purpose.

THE STRATEGIC FAMILY THERAPY ALTERNATIVE

Many psychotherapeutic modalities have been empirically proved to effectively treat emotionally disturbed children. By contrast, antipsychotics can at best mask symptoms in the short term, but the cost of these short-term benefits is staggering. As Whitaker documents in chapter 1, antipsychotics cause significant harm to children's developing brains and bodies. Of equal concern, medicalizing children's psychological suffering prevents families from seeking the help that they need to effect meaningful personal, interpersonal, and cultural change and growth.

As recently as 1990, psychotherapy as opposed to drug therapy was the treatment of choice for emotionally disturbed children, and empirical research continues to support its efficacy. In my bid to restore psychotherapy to its rightful place within the mental health system, I will focus on the approach that I use in my clinical work: strategic family therapy (SFT) as developed by Jay Haley and Cloe Madanes, which is synergistic with the concepts of symbolic anthropology as elucidated by Victor and Edith Turner. Strategic family therapy is a *social therapy* in that it locates the child's problems in the relationships among family members—not in the child—and it avoids the pitfalls of medicalization. I close the chapter with a clinical case vignette of an adolescent who was becoming violent at home and school and who narrowly averted a course of antipsychotic medication. In the sections that follow, I provide an overview of the theoretical foundation of SFT. I believe that rites of passage and cybernetic processes are at the heart of the therapeutic value of SFT, and I elucidate these concepts below.

RITES OF PASSAGE, PSYCHOTHERAPY, AND SOCIAL TRANSITION

Rites of passage are ritual events that serve to move a person from one social status to another—for example from childhood to adulthood and from illness to health—by reordering social relations within the group. Rites of passage have been discovered in every known society since the beginning of recorded history, and this underscores their essential role in the development and transformation of human identity.

A century ago, the French anthropologist Arnold van Gennep formulated *Les Rites de Passage*.[8] His theory provides an elegant description of the continuity of human life as the ordering and reordering of social relations through ritual. He maintained the following:

1. Human life is a series of transitions through well-defined social positions; this is a symbolic journey through social time and space.
2. Transition is disturbing to the individual and society.
3. Ritual cushions the disturbing effect of transition on the individual *and* the society.

Van Gennep unified what appeared to be a diverse class of cultural rituals by demonstrating that they share the same purpose and structure. Rituals accompany changes in the social status or activity of individuals and groups, such as birth, marriage, illness, and death. They all share the same three-stage symbolic structure, which he called "the pattern of the rites of passage":

1. Separation: participants are symbolically separated from everyday life; death of the old status.

2. *Limen* (German for "threshold"): doorway into space where new status is symbolically conceived.

3. Reincorporation: participants are symbolically reborn into everyday life in a new status.

I would argue that all forms of healing, including psychotherapy and even Western medicine, share this symbolic structure or "pattern of the rites of passage."

Cybernetic Theory

The development of cybernetic theory in 1948 had a profound effect on science in general and on behavioral science in particular.[9] Enlightenment science divided, labeled, and categorized people, things, and events as discreet entities. While medical illness may be adequately addressed by studying biological processes within the individual, this narrow focus is inadequate for analyzing or intervening in the meanings generated by and shared between two or more people. Cybernetic theory shifted the unit of analysis from objects, people, and events, to the *information carried* by objects, people, and events in a system.

The cybernetic unit of analysis and intervention is a system defined as: INPUT→PROCESS→OUTPUT. A portion of the information contained in the output is fed back into the system, creating a homeostatic, or self-regulating feedback loop. Positive feedback amplifies or increases the output, while negative feedback dampens or reduces output. A system that receives only positive feedback will produce more and more of the same output until it eventually breaks down, whereas a system that receives only negative feedback will produce less and less output until it eventually stops altogether.

Cybernetic ideas help us to conceptualize social organizations, like a village or a family, as self-correcting systems that encourage stability. Children's behavioral issues when understood systemically play a vital role in reestablishing homeostasis within a family that is no longer functioning productively.

A Successful Model of Health Care

Victor and Edith Turner's research on healing rituals provides a penetrating analysis of the role of both ritual and cybernetics in healing individuals and groups. In the early 1950s, they studied the Ndembu who live in small villages in northwestern Zambia. The Turners observed,

"As we became increasingly part of the village scene, we discovered that very often decisions to perform rituals were connected with crises in the social life of the village."[10] When social conflict was high, one of its members—an innocent third party, *often a child*—was afflicted with an illness. The Ndembu believed that illness is caused by spirit possession, which requires a village healing ritual to remove the spirit, and that death is the result of quarrels among the living. In order to heal the afflicted person, village adversaries felt it necessary to collaborate with each other in order to conduct a ritual that exorcises the possessing spirit, and this intense shared experience also served to heal their adversarial relationships. These observations led Victor Turner to conclude that the spirit being drawn out of the afflicted person really represented the hidden animosities of the village.[11] In Van Gennep's words, ritual changes or reorders social relations; the old conflicting relationships "die," and cooperative relations are "reborn" or reestablished. Thus, both the individual and society undergo healthy change.

The Turners suggested that the healing rituals that restored the social well-being of the village can also be understood in the language of cybernetics. Conflict in village social life was a form of positive feedback that would lead to progressively more conflict and eventually destroy the village if left unchecked. An individual became afflicted in response to the level of social conflict in the village, which created a crisis that in turn triggered a ritual. Ritual served as a form of negative feedback, which lessened the conflict and restored normal relations among the villagers by obligating them to cooperate in order to heal the afflicted individual.

After Victor's untimely death in 1980, Edith returned to Zambia to revisit their research on the Ndembu's healing rituals. Upon her return to the United States, she was delighted to share with me, "Their rituals have gotten better. They are curing more people." Surprised by this discovery, I asked her why this was. She responded, "In 1953 they tried to cure everything with ritual. Since then they have learned to send the TB cases to the hospital and cure the rest with ritual."[12] To which I responded, "During that same time, we have learned to send everything to the hospital." Ironically, the Ndembu who believe in spirit possession, can discriminate between a disease and a behavioral problem and treat each accordingly, while here in the West, our embrace of the narrative of medical progress leads us to see all problems as diseases requiring medical intervention with disastrous results.

The Turners' work illuminates one of the great ironies of Western civilization: the same World War II science that created cybernetic theory also created Thorazine—the first antipsychotic—an event that launched the dominance of the medical model in psychiatry. At the very moment that cybernetics created a framework for a deeper and more complex understanding of human nature, the medicalization of psychiatry forestalled its application. As a result, millions of children have suffered from the iatrogenic consequences of unnecessary and dangerous drug use, while being denied meaningful psychotherapeutic intervention.

Medication versus Psychotherapy: Ceremony versus Ritual

Victor Turner made a critical distinction between *rituals* that accompany a rite of passage, which *transform* an individual's status, versus *ceremonies* that *reaffirm* an existing status. Psychotherapy can be likened to a ritual that transforms one's status, for example, from that of mentally ill to healthy. In contrast, the act of prescribing a psychiatric drug can be compared to a ceremony that symbolizes and thereby makes visible a person's alleged mental illness. The individual then risks becoming frozen in his or her status of mentally ill rather than being transported to the status of healthy.

For the last 50 years, it has been assumed that the modern psychiatric narrative of chemical imbalance was reducing the social stigma of mental illness. However, new research shows that this has not been the case. In fact, the chemical imbalance narrative has actually been increasing stigma. Perhaps knowing that a person takes an antipsychotic encourages others to treat that individual more harshly and locks the individual into the status of chronic mental patient. The symbolic impact of the drug prescription may in fact be playing a significant role in the dramatic increase in chronic mental illness since antipsychotics were first introduced.

Strategic Family Therapy: A Creative Synthesis of Cybernetics and Rites of Passage

Strategic family therapy, which grew out of cybernetic thinking, conceptualizes the presenting child's emotional distress or behavioral issues as serving a corrective to an unhealthy family system. Strategic family therapists believe that two kinds of triads with dysfunctional coalitions cause the lion's share of problems within families: (1) a two-generation coalition and (2) a three-generation coalition. In a two-generation coalition, a parent (or member of the parental generation) joins a child against another member of the parental generation. If the coalition is secret or covert, the child's problem is likely to be more serious. Whether coalitions are explicit or covert, they are an observable, patterned behavior. For example, in a two-generation problem, a father might say to his son, "It is 8:30 and time for bed"; the mother might overtly challenge father's authority by stating, "Oh, it's too early for him to turn in," or speak to her son directly, "It's too early, so you don't have to go right now." In a covert coalition, the mother might simply roll her eyes or wink at her son, indicating he doesn't have to comply with father's instructions. In a three-generation coalition, a grandparent (usually a grandmother) joins a grandchild against the parental generation in the middle (usually a single mother). The grandmother acts overtly or covertly in ways that countermand the mother's authority, and the mother becomes like a sister to her child.

Cybernetic thinking understands a child's problem as a particular type of behavior that has been adopted as a corrective to or as a form of protection from dysfunction within the family.[13] From this perspective, the problem does not reside within the child; rather, the problem is a maladaptive sequence of behaviors among family members. The target of therapeutic change is the problem sequence rather than a particular person in the sequence. Therefore, it is pointless, as well as harmful, to drug *any* of the participants in the sequence. Here is an example of a maladaptive repeating sequence: (1) Two parents quarrel. (2) In response, their child develops a problem. (3) The child's problem creates a crisis that forces the parents to set their own issues aside and deal with their child. (4) The parents respond by pulling together. (5) When they pull together, the child behaves. (6) When the child behaves, the parents disagree again, which returns the family to step 1, and the problem sequence repeats. Understanding the child's behavior within this larger context makes it evident that the child is actually trying to fix a problem within the family, and addressing the child's behavior as if it *is* the problem misses the bigger picture. A strategic family therapist conceptualizes the problem at the level of the family and attempts to reorganize the family structure so that the child no longer needs to act out.

Strategic family therapy transforms the sequence as follows: (1) The child's crisis brings the family to therapy. (2) The therapist empowers the parents to take charge of and solve their child's problem. (3) As they cooperate to solve the child's problem, (4) their own relationship is transformed—and their fighting stops—(5) the child's problem stops, and the cycle of trouble is broken. (6) The family does not go back to step 1, because the parents' relationship is strengthened and the child no longer needs to act out in order to bring the parents into harmony.

By contrast, when a mental health professional medicalizes the child's problem, it prevents the reorganization of the family system that leads to growth and instead the following ensues: (1) Two parents quarrel. (2) Their child develops a problem and is brought for treatment to a mental health professional who diagnoses him or her. (3) The doctor tries to fix the problem with a drug prescription. (4) The parents are not involved in the solution in a meaningful way, their relationship does not change, and they do not move to the next stage of the family life cycle. (5) The child is temporarily quieted by the sedating effects of drugs, rather than from substantive changes in family organization. (6) The parents quarrel again, and the sequence repeats, but in step 3, the doctor may continue to experiment with a stronger dose, a different drug, or multiple drugs to fix the child. The drug has an iatrogenic effect on the child, while also preventing healthy growth and change within the family.

A medicalized problem sequence is comparable to the vicious cycle described by Rachel Carson in *Silent Spring*. The initial application of DDT was meant to target a particular type of insect but instead killed many species of insect, causing a variety of insect-eating birds to starve to death. The next year, there were even more insects and fewer birds—so *more* DDT was used. The more heavily DDT was applied, the more damaged the ecological niche became. Similarly, when psychiatric drugs are used to address a child's maladaptive behavior, the child's ecological niche, or family system, is further damaged, and appropriate intervention in the form of psychotherapy is forestalled, leading to a heavier drug prescription or more drugs causing still more damage.

Psychiatry assumes that a child's psychological issues are biological events that have no meaning and sweeps the important social and contextual information that is being conveyed under the rug of genetic malfunction. In contrast, SFT assumes that the child's difficulties signify that the family is having trouble making a needed life cycle change, and furthermore, they serve as metaphors that describe the nature of the family's dysfunction.

THE NATURAL BORN KILLER: A CASE STUDY

When I first met Peter, he was a 17-year-old high school sophomore in a special education program for emotionally disturbed youth, who lived with his single mother, Kris, and his 19-year-old sister, Karen. Shortly before our first session, a staff member at his school had recommended a course of antipsychotics because of his impulsive and violent behavior. A colleague of mine who worked at the school and was familiar with my approach to family therapy referred Peter to my clinic in the hope of averting the drug prescription.

In my first session with the family, I learned that Kris was a dedicated and hardworking single mother whose partner and the father of
her two children had abandoned the family when the children were
still toddlers. Kris's working-class parents, Frank and Jean, were very
involved in Peter and Karen's upbringing. Kris had one sibling, an
overachiever who had graduated from college, was married to a professional man, and had two children who were straight-A students
bound for prestigious universities. Jean frequently held Kris's sister
out to her as a yardstick with which to measure her failures. Kris, by
contrast with her sister, was a never-married single mother whose son
was emotionally disturbed and whose daughter was a high school
dropout with a history of unstable relationships with boyfriends. The
previous year, Karen ran away from home with a boy from another
state. She had recently returned home after the relationship failed
and had immediately entered into another chaotic relationship. Since
returning home, she had made no effort to find work and was fully
dependent on her mother who had vehemently disapproved of her
dropping out of school. Based on my observations during the first session, I surmised that the family was locked into a three-generation coalition in which Peter and Karen's grandmother, Jean, had assumed
the role of the mother, relegating Kris to the status of sister and thus
preventing her from disciplining her children effectively. My second
session with the family confirmed this supposition.

The day after my first meeting with the family, Kris called me in a
state of panic, and I got a taste of how volatile the family system was.
Peter had threatened to kill his sister, Karen. When Karen took refuge
in the bathroom, he plunged a large butcher's knife through the door
and stormed out of the apartment. I advised Kris to call the police and
have Peter taken into custody, and I arranged for an emergency session
with the family the next day. Peter was removed to a detention center
where I knew the personnel who trusted my judgment regarding the
timing of his release.

During the second session, which took place in Peter's absence because he was still being held at the detention center, Karen provided
more details about the circumstances surrounding the assault. Peter
had attacked her after she had been out all night with her boyfriend.
Guided by information that Karen had disclosed earlier in the session, and without condoning Peter's behavior, I explored the possibility that his conduct was not simply that of a crazy person, but rather
that it was a meaningful communication in response to her behavior. I asked Karen whether it was possible that Peter was disturbed
by the fact that she wasn't working and was burdening her mother.
Peter's grandfather Frank immediately and vigorously affirmed this

suggestion, asserting that Peter was not only upset by Karen's failure to look for work but also by her turbulent relationship with her boyfriend because he worried that his mother was working too hard and was overwhelmed. Karen responded by stating that she often felt that she needed to answer to Peter and that when she didn't meet his demands or expectations, he would become angry and she would become scared. Kris concurred with Karen's description of her relationship with her brother, and Jean added that Peter had been the man of the house for as long as she could remember. From this exchange, a very different picture of Peter began to emerge. Rather than Peter the crazy person, he was portrayed by his family as an adolescent who from early childhood had struggled under the weight of the responsibility that he felt to be the man of the house. By taking on this role, it robbed him of his mother who was transformed into a weak sibling who needed his protection, it strained his relationship with Karen, and it encouraged Karen to treat her mother like a peer rather than an authority figure. In consequence, Karen played the rebellious daughter to Peter's incompetent father, and Kris became the sister that she could blithely disobey. Kris's status of sibling was further cemented by Jean's portrait of Kris as an incompetent failure. It was clear at this point that my work as a therapist was to facilitate transformations in status that would enable Kris to reclaim her role as mother, Jean as grandmother, and Peter and Karen as healthy children. If instead, as had been originally recommended, Peter had been given antipsychotics, it would have reified his status of emotionally disturbed and blocked family members from shedding their dysfunctional statuses and acquiring new ones.

In spite of the fact that everyone in the family was able to identify Peter's struggle to be man of the house,. I quickly learned that they were more deeply invested in his status of crazy person, and Jean immediately began to push back as soon as this status was challenged. Soon after Frank described Peter's protective stance toward his mother, Jean interjected: "Peter doesn't understand all the terrible things he does . . . [because] he goes crazy." At this point, all the others, Kris, Karen, and Frank, vigorously agreed with Jean's definition of Peter as crazy. Frank further entrenched the family myth by suggesting that Peter had in fact been a disturbed child from birth. In Frank's words, "He's been that way all his life." He then retold an episode that occurred when Peter was 4 or 5 years old; he jumped on his mother's back and said, "Mommy I'm going to kill you!" Everyone in the family rallied around this depiction of Peter's natural, lifelong desire to hurt others. Jean added icing to the cake when she said, "He seems to take joy in hurting others. And as soon as he's finished and he knows he has hurt you, then he wants to put his arms around you and love you." These comments betrayed the family's deeply held conviction that Peter was mentally ill and therefore had no control over his violent impulses as well as their resistance to the competing notion that his behavior was meaningful.

In the same session, Jean further asserted her status as "mother" and her belief that Kris was incompetent with the comment that "When [Peter] is with me, he is fine. He's so passive. He's just beautiful. But I can see the anger building up, even before he leaves me . . . when he is going home . . ."

We see in this family script, no doubt endlessly rehearsed day after day and year after year, how individual identity is created, assigned, and maintained by joint participation in a repeating sequence of acts. From a cybernetic perspective, the family consensus that Peter was crazy served as positive feedback that was further destabilizing the family system, which was at risk of being destroyed. While destruction of a family can take many forms, in this case it was likely that left unchecked, Peter's behavior would have led to a career as a mental patient or a criminal, and the family would have stabilized around that tragedy.

In my role as a strategic family therapist, I helped to catalyze a series of role reassignments: Jean and Frank would become real grandparents instead of superparents, Kris would be mother instead of sister, Peter would no longer have to serve as a father figure, and this would free Peter and Karen from their destructive patterns of behavior. In order to engender these changes in status within the family, I needed to establish their commitment to the process. I asked for their promise to call the police if Peter became violent again. I recognized that calling the police on their beloved son and grandson was traumatic and that it would play a powerful role in their commitment to making deep and lasting changes. I then asked Kris to draw up an explicit set of rules with escalating consequences for escalating behaviors for both Peter and Karen, in the process, reinstating her status as parent rather than sibling. Jean and Frank were asked to serve an advisory role more appropriate to their status as grandparents. Toward the end of the second session, I escorted the family to the detention center, where Kris presented the basic framework of rules to Peter in the presence of the others. Peter agreed to follow the new rules and also to sign an agreement the next day as a condition of his release.

When I met with Peter's family shortly before he was discharged the next day, it was evident that the status transformations that I had initiated were already beginning to take hold. Karen came to the session dressed professionally in a neatly ironed blouse and slacks in sharp contrast to the tank top and miniskirt she had worn to the previous session. I learned that her mother had secured a position for her at her place of work and Karen had accepted it. Quite literally overnight, she had metamorphosed from a rebellious teen to a responsible youth. With her own parents relegated to a supporting role, Kris presented her carefully worked out set of rules with escalating consequences for escalating transgressions to Peter and the rest of the family. Through this exercise, Kris had begun to reclaim her rightful status as mother. Another significant shift that was revealed in this third session was that Kris, Jean, and Frank were able to acknowledge Peter's strengths—his generosity, his ability to take responsibility, and his capacity for altruism—thus moving away from their investment in his status as insane.

During my fourth meeting with the family a week later, we discussed the fact that at the rate that he was proceeding through school, Peter would be 21 before graduating from high school. Peter and his family agreed that it would be more productive for him to find a full-time job and work toward his GED. Peter found a job within a week, and the family was so significantly improved that I terminated the therapy after one more session.

An eight-month phone follow-up with Kris revealed that the changes in the family were stable. Peter expressed that he was glad to be out of trouble. He acknowledged that there were family problems at times, but these were settled by talking and not by getting angry or throwing things. He stopped having fits and enjoyed working, he got his driver's license, and he completed his GED six months after the last session. Karen remained gainfully employed as well.

I believe the long-term success of this case followed from the initial reorganization of the family leadership around the crisis created by Peter's detention; when Peter was released, he entered a new family organization in which Kris's corrected status gave her appropriate authority over her children, and Jean and Frank assumed their rightful status as grandparents, rather than parents. When Kris, with the support of her own parents, could treat Peter and Karen as responsible children, they responded as responsible children.

CONCLUSION

This case example is illustrative of my work with children who under most circumstances would end up drugged and incarcerated. By understanding and treating the problems of each child and youth as a unique social agreement among persons who care for and love each other, and by understanding that while problem behaviors can have devastating consequences, they also have purpose and meaning for the families in which they occur, the stage is then set for meaningful therapeutic work. When a family is approached with these understandings, chances are good that they will actively participate in resolving their own problems without psychiatric drugs. There is more evidence that mental illness is a social construct—a social status—rather than a physical disease and a significant body of research to support the efficacy of psychotherapy.

The status of children in our consumer society has changed. Children are no longer forced to labor endlessly in sweatshops that *produce things.* Their new work is to *consume things.* Anyone's child will do as a consumer, even when it means consuming dangerous, life-shortening drugs. American children are now forced to consume drugs that are just as damaging to their minds, their bodies, and their lives as the spinning belts and gears of 19th-century machinery on which they were once forced to labor. Hopefully, by highlighting the problems of medicalizing childhood, I have helped to create a crisis that will trigger a healing ritual in my own village.

9

How Parents Can Improve Their Children's Developmental Trajectories

Adena B. Meyers and Laura E. Berk

Over the past 15 years, the number of children hospitalized for psychiatric reasons and the numbers receiving various psychiatric diagnoses indicative of disruptive and potentially dangerous behavior increased dramatically. For instance, between 1996 and 2007, psychiatric hospitalizations among children under age 14 nearly doubled, and the rate among adolescents increased by more than 40 percent.[1] Meanwhile, rates of attention-deficit/hyperactivity disorder (ADHD) diagnoses increased by about 3 percent per year between 1997 and 2006, reaching a prevalence of nearly one in ten children aged 4 to 17 by 2007.[2] In addition, autism spectrum disorder diagnoses increased by more than 50 percent between 2002 and 2006 to an average of 9 cases per 1,000 eight-year-olds.[3] Perhaps the most startling of these recent trends concerns the sharp increase in bipolar disorder (BD) diagnoses among children. Compared to the mid-1990s, children seen in outpatient settings in 2002–2003 were *40 times* more likely to be diagnosed with BD.[4] This latter development likely reflects a range of factors—including a considerable number of misdiagnoses—but nevertheless reveals that increasing numbers of children are presenting with behavior patterns that are extremely troubling to those around them. It has also lead to an increasing use of pharmacotherapy in treating children's mental health problems,[5] as more than 90 percent of children seen for BD receive some form of psychotropic medication.[6]

Although there are undoubtedly numerous reasons for the increases in psychiatric diagnosis and use of pharmacotherapy in children, one factor that may be contributing to these trends is a growing sense among parents that their child-rearing responsibilities are overwhelming, and their efforts to positively influence their children's development are inadequate. For instance, a nationally representative survey of more than 1,600 parents revealed that 61 percent were critical of their own efforts—that is, judged the job that they were doing in rearing their children as either "fair" or "poor." More than half believed that parents of previous generations did better.[7] Results of another large, nationally representative survey indicate that between 1997 and 2002, the percent of parents reporting that their children "are much harder to care for than most" or "do things that bother them a lot" increased by 50 percent from 6 to 9 percent,[8] reflecting a belief among some parents that their children's behavior is becoming increasingly difficult to manage.

As a result, many of today's parents need and want help to better understand and address their children's challenging behavior, and it is not surprising that they are turning to family doctors, pediatricians, psychiatrists, psychologists, and other mental health specialists for this assistance. Practitioners trained within the medical model are likely to approach diagnosis and classification of mental health problems by applying categorical labels from the *Diagnostic and Statistical Manual of Mental Disorders* (*DSM*) to children's emotional and behavioral difficulties. Moreover, third-party payers require providers to use this diagnostic system in order to receive reimbursement for their services. Unfortunately, although these diagnostic labels are helpful for communication among professionals, and provide some utility for selecting treatments, they offer little help to parents who want to know how they can be part of the solution—that is, what they can do in their role as parents to improve their children's current and future functioning.

As critics of this system have pointed out, the *DSM* creates labels for diagnostic categories that were originally developed as hypothetical constructs describing mental health problems primarily seen in adults. Some consider the diagnostic criteria to be problematic, especially when applied to children, because of their focus on current symptoms and behavior outside of any developmental context. Little attention is paid to the many risk and protective factors that may influence children's trajectories over time. Instead, there is a tendency to reify diagnostic labels while losing sight of their hypothetical nature. This may create the erroneous impression that a tangible disease entity with known causes, processes, and treatment mechanisms permanently resides within each affected child.[9]

As evidence mounts regarding genetic and neuropsychological causes and correlates of various mental health problems,[10] there is a certain appeal to this medical conceptualization. And the idea of treating these conditions at a biological level, with medications that may reverse or cure the underlying disease, seems a logical corollary. There are several problems with this view, however. First, although psychotropic medications are effective in reducing some psychiatric symptoms,[11] they generally have not been shown to reverse disease processes. We simply do not know enough about the causal mechanisms of most mental health problems or the processes mediating effective treatments to make such strong claims. Second, there is ample evidence that psychosocial processes and interventions can improve outcomes for children experiencing a host of developmental and mental health problems. As we will illustrate in this chapter, these psychosocial factors often involve parents. Indeed, parents profoundly influence development and thus can play a central role in enhancing their children's current and future functioning.

DEVELOPMENTAL PSYCHOPATHOLOGY AND PARENTS' ROLE IN SHAPING CHILDREN'S TRAJECTORIES

In contrast to the categorical diagnostic system exemplified by the *DSM*, a perspective know as *developmental psychopathology* provides an alternative conceptualization of children's emotional and behavioral difficulties in which the effects of key developmental influences, including parents, play a more prominent role. Instead of focusing on current symptoms, this approach considers adaptive and maladaptive behavior in developmental context. It emphasizes risk and protective factors within the child, family, and broader environment, and assumes that variables at each of these levels may alter (for better or worse) the course of development.[12] This implies that development is malleable—that as risk and protective factors change over time, so does the course of development, so that a child exhibiting signs of maladaptive functioning at one point may show improvements later if risks diminish or protective factors increase. By the same token, a high-functioning child may later encounter developmental challenges or stressors that adversely affect outcomes.

Multifinality and *equifinality*, two key concepts borrowed from systems theory, are used in the developmental psychopathology literature to illustrate these divergent developmental possibilities.[13] Multifinality describes situations in which a single starting point may lead to an array of different outcomes, whereas equifinality refers to the possibility that individuals may arrive at a common outcome from a variety of different starting points. Paul Frick and Essi Viding recently illustrated how these concepts may be applied to research findings related to the development of antisocial behavior. For example, fearless and uninhibited temperament places children at risk for developing callous traits, low empathy, and antisocial behavior. However, in the presence of other individual characteristics and socialization experiences (including parental warmth and consistent, obedience-oriented parental discipline), many uninhibited children successfully internalize social norms about right and wrong, and thus may grow up to be *bold* rather than *mean,* an example of multifinality. On the other hand, antisocial behavior may result from impulsive temperament, verbal deficits, suboptimal parenting, exposure to antisocial models within the peer group, or various combinations of these risk factors, thus exemplifying equifinality.[14] Although parenting is not the only influence on children's development, its potential impact is clear and prominent in these examples.

This discussion is not intended to convey that serious mental health problems in children do not exist, or that their effects can be reversed easily or completely. Parents of children with psychiatric difficulties do face significant child-rearing challenges, and in many cases know that their children are likely to encounter a variety of obstacles throughout childhood and adulthood. Still, even in the case of some of the most severe psychiatric conditions, the developmental psychopathology framework provides a complex, multilevel, dynamic perspective on risk and resilience over the course of development in which long-term outcomes are not set in stone, and parents can make a difference in their children's development.[15]

Consistent with this perspective, research indicates that maternal sensitivity during the toddler years predicts improved expressive language development among young children who are later diagnosed with autism.[16] Among adolescents and adults with this diagnosis, high levels of maternal warmth and praise and low levels of criticism are associated with improved social relationships and reduced internalizing, externalizing, and repetitive behavioral symptoms.[17] These findings illustrate the principle of multifinality, demonstrating variation in the range and severity of presenting problems among individuals with autism, in part as a function of parenting.

Similarly, families of individuals with severe psychotic or mood disorders can influence patterns of adaptation or maladaptation by adjusting their communication patterns with respect to expressed emotion. For example, hospitalization rates of patients with schizophrenia are much higher in families with communication patterns characterized by high levels of criticism or emotional overinvolvement, compared to families with lower levels of these behaviors.[18] Although most work to date in this area has focused on families of adult psychiatric patients, recently a group of researchers experimentally evaluated an intervention targeting expressed emotion and communication patterns in families of adolescents diagnosed with bipolar disorder. Results revealed that over a two-year period, adolescents in the intervention group experienced faster recovery from and less time overall in depressive episodes compared to adolescents in the control group.[19]

INTERACTIONS AMONG GENETIC PREDISPOSITIONS AND PARENTING INFLUENCES

The developmental psychopathology perspective, and the concepts of multifinality and equifinality underscore the complexity of developmental trajectories, in which even the most salient variables never operate in isolation. Developmental risks do not lead inevitably to deleterious outcomes, and protective factors do not provide failsafe insurance against maladjustment. This complexity is especially evident in results of recent research on the interplay between genetic and environmental influences on adaptive and maladaptive development. The findings demonstrate that genetic factors play an important role in the development and course of psychopathology, but their influence is rarely direct or simple. Indeed, although research on genetics may seem to support a medical conceptualization of mental health and mental illness, results reveal that genetic predispositions interact with socialization factors in ways that clearly illustrate the principles of developmental psychopathology, highlighting parents' potential to influence child development.

Heritability evidence, based on comparisons of identical and fraternal twins, indicates that genetic influences on temperamental traits that place children at risk for psychopathology (activity level, attention span, irritability, and behavioral dysregulation) are moderate, with about half of individual differences among children attributed to their genetic make-up.[20] Similarly, with respect to diagnosed childhood disorders (with the exception of ADHD, for which heritability estimates tend to be higher) modest heritabilities have been obtained for children's internalizing and externalizing disorders, including anxiety and conduct problems.[21] Genetics, of course, influences *all behavior* to some degree, making the heritabilities just reported unsurprising. Nevertheless, because twin samples seriously underestimate environmental variation in the general child population—and often do not adequately represent the high-risk environments known to be associated with psychopathology—heritability findings are believed to exaggerate genetic effects.[22] Consequently, even high heritability estimates leave plenty of room for environmental influences (including parenting) to play significant roles in developmental outcomes.

Indeed, it is frequently impossible to separate genetic and parenting risks for childhood disorders because they tend to be correlated: Genetically influenced mental disorders are linked to high-risk home environments that heighten susceptibility to psychopathology. Many studies confirm that mentally ill parents are more likely to create family contexts characterized by discord, diminished warmth and child involvement, as well as punitive and inconsistent discipline—factors strongly predictive of serious, lasting mental health problems in children.[23] Furthermore, children with difficult temperamental traits (intense, negative emotional reactivity; poor adaptability to unfamiliar experiences) often evoke maladaptive parenting. As infants, they are less likely to receive warm, sensitive caregiving, and by the second year, their parents tend to resort to angry, punitive, and inconsistent discipline—practices that heighten the child's irritable, conflict-ridden style.[24]

Yet research also verifies that uncoupling unfavorable gene-environment correlations by providing genetically vulnerable children with positive child-rearing experiences often yields good adjustment, confirming the vital role of parenting in children's developmental trajectories. For example, when parents are warm and sensitive, which helps infants and toddlers regulate negative emotion, temperamental difficulty declines by ages two to three.[25] In toddlerhood and childhood, parental sensitivity, support, clear expectations, and limit-setting foster self-regulation, reducing the likelihood that difficult temperament will persist and lead to emotional and social difficulties.[26] A large Finnish adoption study illustrates the impact of such uncoupling of gene-environment correlations with respect to psychopathology: Children whose biological mothers had schizophrenia but who were being reared by healthy adoptive parents showed little mental illness—no more than a control group with healthy biological and adoptive parents. In contrast, schizophrenia and other psychological disorders piled up in adoptees whose biological and adoptive parents were both disturbed.[27] These examples illustrate the principle of multifinality, demonstrating that the long-term effects of risk factors such as difficult temperament and maternal schizophrenia are not always stable, and that parenting can alter the developmental course for youngsters who start out life with various vulnerabilities.

The positive heritability evidence summarized earlier has spurred researchers to begin searching for specific genes that place children at risk for psychopathology. The genetic markers detected to date account for only a small proportion of the wide variation in children's temperamental styles and only a minority of cases of psychological disorders.[28] Yet identification of these genotypes has opened the door to more precise studies of the impact of parenting on children at high genetic risk for psychological disorders. The efforts are uncovering provocative *gene-environment interactions*—meaning that certain children, because of their genetic makeup, respond uniquely to parenting experiences.

Together, the investigations convey a consistent theme, further illustrating the principles of equifinality and multifinality: Temperamentally difficult children function much worse than other children when exposed to inept parenting, yet benefit most from good parenting. One study focused on 2-year-olds with a chromosome-17 gene containing a certain repetition of DNA base pairs (called short 5-HTTLPR), which interferes with functioning of the inhibitory neurotransmitter serotonin and, thus, greatly increases the risk of emotional reactivity and self-regulation difficulties. Children with this gene became increasingly irritable and dysregulated as their mothers' anxiety about parenting increased, whereas maternal anxiety had little impact on children without this genetic marker.[29] In another investigation, preschoolers with the short 5-HTTLPR gene responded especially strongly to positive parenting. With parental affection and support, their capacity for self-regulation equaled that of agemates with a low-risk genotype.

Other studies have focused on several genes that alter functioning of the neurotransmitter dopamine (involved in motivation and reward), thereby increasing children's risk of deficient inhibition, ADHD, and externalizing behavior problems. In one investigation, children with one of these markers (a chromosome-11 gene with a special DNA base-pair repeat, labeled DRD4 7-repeat) who had insensitive mothers displayed more externalizing problems than children without the gene, irrespective of their mothers' sensitivity. At the same time, children with the DRD4 7-repeat gene and sensitive mothers exhibited the lowest levels of externalizing problems![30] Investigations of other dopamine-related genes reveal similar effects for children with high-risk genotypes: greater behavioral disturbance than their counterparts in the presence of adverse child-rearing, yet greater responsiveness to positive child-rearing.[31]

In sum, new evidence indicates that children with certain genotypes are especially susceptible to parenting effects. In the face of poor
parenting, their development suffers much more than that of other
children. Yet these children also respond more strongly to the devel-
opment-enhancing impact of supportive parenting, in some instances
exceeding their counterparts without genetic risks in favorable adjustment. For parents of young children with challenging temperamental
traits and behaviors, news of these findings can be empowering. Although such parents face challenging parenting tasks, the very child
characteristics that require increased parental effort and investment
may also make parenting more potent and influential.

AUTHORITATIVE STYLE: THE FUNDAMENTALS
OF GOOD PARENTING

In the studies just reported, and in countless others documenting the
relationship of parenting to concurrent and future child outcomes, the
features of good parenting are similar. Together, they form the authoritative child-rearing style, a combination of three categories of parenting behaviors that, when implemented over a wide range of situations,
generate an enduring, positive child-rearing climate with numerous
protective benefits.[32] These ingredients are:

1. *Acceptance and involvement.* Authoritative parents are warm, attentive, and sensitive to their child's needs. They take time to establish an enjoyable, emotionally fulfilling bond that draws their child into close connection. This affectionate,
   caring relationship motivates children—even those who are temperamentally
   inattentive, impulsive, and difficult to rear[33]—to listen to and follow parents'
   suggestions and directives, as a means of preserving a gratifying parent-child tie.
2. *Control.* Authoritative parents exercise firm, reasonable control. They consistently
   insist on mature behavior, enforce their demands, and give age-appropriate reasons for their expectations. By offering explanations, authoritative parents exert
   control in ways that appear to the child as fair and reasonable, not arbitrary,
   thereby inducing far more compliance, as well as personal adoption of parental
   standards, than other child management strategies.
3. *Autonomy granting.* Authoritative parents engage in gradual, appropriate autonomy granting, allowing the child to make decisions in areas where he or she is
   ready to make choices. Their goal is to nurture a responsible, mature young person. Because authoritative parents are firm and rational early on, they earn the
   privilege of easing up later, because their children have developed self-control.

Protective Benefits of Authoritative Parenting

Many studies show that these fundamentals of good parenting promote all the elements that describe a well-adjusted child: an upbeat
mood, empathy, kindness, honesty, cooperativeness, positive social

skills, motivation to learn, and good school performance. Furthermore, authoritative parenting deters emotional and behavior problems. And it is effective for children of both genders and of diverse ages, temperaments, and socioeconomic backgrounds.[34] The authoritative style also has broad cultural validity, predicting cognitive and social competence across many ethnic groups and in cultures as different from the United States as China and Korea.[35] Indeed, most cultures sense the value of authoritative parenting. A survey of parenting in more than 180 societies found that a combination of warmth and reasonable control is the most common pattern of child-rearing around the world.[36]

Because many forces in addition to parents play a role in children's upbringing, implementing the authoritative style does not ensure a problem-free child. But children whose parents are authoritative are far more likely to develop in healthy ways and far less likely to have serious difficulties than children of parents who use other approaches. Indeed, supportive aspects of the authoritative style are a powerful source of resilience, helping children surmount biologically based limitations and protecting them from the negative impact of family stress and other environmental threats to development.[37]

PARENTS AS PART OF THE SOLUTION: EVIDENCE-BASED PARENTING STRATEGIES AND INTERVENTIONS

Although the authoritative style provides a general blueprint for positive parenting, those who adopt this style have a number of choices to consider, and may confront various challenges and obstacles as they navigate their child-rearing responsibilities. Below we elaborate on several of these parenting issues some of which pertain to all families, others of which affect only particular subgroups. Universally relevant parenting issues include choices about discipline practices, management of children's peer relations, and responses to children's emotional experiences and expressions. More specific topics include parenting challenges related to parental mental health and divorce. As we will see, parents have considerable potential to influence their children's developmental trajectories through their decisions and actions in each of these domains. In addition, evidence-based interventions exist that may help promote optimal parenting practices in each area.

Discipline Practices: Effective Methods of Control

In their efforts to exercise firm and reasonable control, authoritative parents must select and implement effective, age-appropriate discipline practices. Unfortunately, although many parents are aware that yelling at, slapping, and spanking incites impulsiveness, anger, and hostility in children, physical punishment in the United States is widespread. In a survey of a nationally representative sample of American households, more than half of parents of infants through 12-year-olds reported using corporal punishment. And between ages 3 and 7, when physical punishment of children was highest, more than 80 percent of parents admitted one or more instances of it in the previous year. Moreover, many American parents do not limit themselves to a slap or a spank; more than one-fourth of physically punishing parents said they used a hard object to hit their child,[38] and a wealth of evidence indicates that corporal punishment and physical abuse of children are closely linked.[39] Research confirms that the more physical punishment children experience, the more likely they are to develop serious, lasting mental health problems, in the form of poor academic performance, depression, and antisocial behavior during childhood and adolescence, and criminality, depressive and alcoholic symptoms, and partner and child abuse in adulthood.[40] Thus, one way for parents to help their children develop optimally is to reduce or ideally, eliminate the use of physical punishment from their discipline repertoires.

For many parents this may be more easily said than done, especially if they are not aware of or skilled in the use of alternative discipline methods, or unable, because of high family stress, to implement those methods. Although corporal punishment spans the socioeconomic spectrum, its frequency and harshness are elevated among less educated, economically disadvantaged parents.[41] Furthermore, parents with mental health problems (who are emotionally reactive, depressed, or aggressive) and with conflict-ridden marriages are more likely to be punitive and also to have hard-to manage children, whose disobedience often evokes more parental harshness.[42]

Fortunately, much is known about the elements of effective discipline, and a number of carefully evaluated parent training interventions exist that have been shown to be effective in helping parents of children of various ages and backgrounds to establish authoritative control without resorting to physical punishment.[43] Based on the assumption that the foundation of effective discipline is a warm and supportive parent-child relationship, many evidence-based parent training programs begin by teaching parents strategies they can use to improve their relationships with their children.[44] Building a mutually respectful bond with the child, letting the child know in advance how to act, and praising mature behavior is highly effective. It yields firm conscience development, including empathy after transgressions, responsible behavior, fair play in games with peers, and considerateness of others.[45] Parent-child closeness is very effective: it leads children to heed parental demands because children feel a sense of commitment to the relationship.

In addition, many parent-training programs provide instruction in the use of discipline techniques derived from behavioral and social learning theories. Parents learn to discipline their children by controlling the environmental variables that are known to influence children's behavior. In practice, this means parents can increase compliance and reduce misbehavior through such techniques as stimulus control (e.g., remove from reach/view items that young children are not allowed to play with; anticipate children's needs for rest, food, activities, attention, and routine, and schedule activities accordingly; use clear, developmentally appropriate language when giving commands), positive reinforcement (e.g., encourage desired behavior with praise and attention), differential attention (e.g., attend to children's age-appropriate, desirable behavior and ignore immature, coercive behavior such as whining, defiant talk, and tantrums), and judicious use of nonphysical punishment (e.g., discourage noncompliant or aggressive behavior by applying mildly aversive consequences such as time out or removal of privileges). By consistently using these discipline strategies, parents can provide their children with the benefits of authoritative parenting while avoiding the risks associated with physical punishment.[46]

Parent Management of Peer Relationships

Another key area in which parents can facilitate positive development in their children is in the domain of social skills and peer relationships. Early on, during the preschool years, parents are responsible for managing their youngsters' peer associations. They can help their children develop friendships and adaptive skills by arranging get-togethers and offering guidance on how to enter a peer group, interact with others, solve peer problems, and keep a positive relationship going. All these parental behaviors are associated with children's social skills.[47] Other aspects of parenting also promote children's peer sociability, even when that is not the parents' primary aim. For example, the time parents spend in sensitive, emotionally positive conversations and playing with young children—during which children observe and learn good social skills—is linked to children's social competence.[48]

In adolescence, parents continue to influence young peoples' choice of peers and the quality of their relationships. Teenagers with authoritative parents are more likely to spend time with self-controlled, high-achieving peers, whose attitudes, values, and behaviors further strengthen their maturity. In contrast, adolescents whose parents use less effective child-rearing styles—coercive, permissive, or uninvolved—tend to gravitate toward antisocial, drug-using agemates and to become increasingly like them over time.[49] Recent evidence also demonstrates that secure attachment to and warm interaction with parents predict adolescents' sense of security and positive communication within friendships. Friendship security, in turn, is related to teenagers' sense of security and good communication in dating relationships.[50]

Parents often worry about their children's capacity to resist unfavorable peer pressures during adolescence. But once again, the authoritative style is related to such resistance.[51] Teenagers whose parents are supportive and exert appropriate oversight respect their parents, an attitude that acts as an antidote to negative peer influences.[52] In contrast, adolescents who experience harsh, overbearing parental control or too little control tend to be highly peer oriented, often relying on friends rather than parents for advice about their personal lives and futures and willing to break their parents' rules, ignore their school work, use drugs, engage in early sexual activity, commit delinquent acts, and hide their talents so that they can be popular with agemates.[53]

One important dimension of authoritative control that is particularly important with respect to adolescent peer relations is known as *parental monitoring*. This refers to parents' awareness and supervision of their teenage children's peer relationships. Parents who keep track of where and with whom their adolescents spend their time, who know and communicate with the parents of their teenagers' friends, and who set appropriate limits with respect to socializing (e.g., enforcing curfews, requiring adult supervision at parties), reduce their children's risk for such adverse outcomes as substance use, risky behavior, and delinquency.[54] These findings further underscore the far-reaching benefits of positive parent-child relationships, since monitoring of adolescents is much easier for parents in the context of a cooperative relationship in which the adolescent willingly discloses information: that is, allows the parent to exert oversight.[55] Recent evidence suggests that parental monitoring may be especially beneficial for adolescents who are already at elevated risk of substance use and other maladaptive outcomes due to genetic predispositions[56] or characteristics of their peer relationships.[57] In addition, a number of preventive interventions have been shown to be successful in reducing adolescent problem behavior by increasing parental monitoring.[58]

Responding to Children's Emotions: Parents as Emotion Coaches

John Gottman, a psychologist who has spent decades conducting research on emotion and family processes, coined the term *emotion coaching* to describe an optimal pattern of parent responding to children's emotional experiences and expressions. According to Gottman, "emotion coaching parents" help their children develop emotion regulation skills by providing them with guidance about emotional experience: "Much like athletic coaches, they teach their children strategies to deal with life's ups and downs. They don't object to their children's displays of anger, sadness, or fear. Nor do they ignore them. Instead, they accept negative emotions as a fact of life and they use emotional moments as opportunities for teaching their kids important life lessons and building closer relationships with them."[59] As delineated by Gottman, emotion coaching typically involves five steps: (1) parental awareness of the child's emotion, (2) recognition of the emotion as an opportunity for closeness and guidance, (3) empathic listening and validation of the child's feelings, (4) help with verbally labeling the feelings, (5) exploring problem-solving strategies while setting limits on emotional expression.[60]

Research by Gottman and others demonstrates links between parents' emotion coaching and children's adaptive functioning with respect to emotion regulation, physical health, academic performance, prosocial behavior, and peer relations.[61] In addition, evidence suggests that parent emotion coaching can serve as a source of resilience, buffering children against some of the potentially negative effects of family conflict and divorce.[62] In fact, even when children are exposed to severe conflict and violence within the family, research indicates that both mothers and fathers can serve as emotion coaches, protecting their children from some of the negative emotional and behavioral consequences of growing up within these deleterious environments.[63]

Recently, researchers in Australia developed and evaluated a parenting intervention based on the five steps of emotion coaching just described. Sixty-one preschools were randomly assigned to intervention and wait-list control conditions, and parents of children attending both groups of schools were recruited to participate in the study. The intervention group included 106 parents who received the intervention right away, whereas the control group included 110 parents scheduled to receive the intervention 10 months later. The intervention was delivered to groups of parents in weekly two-hour sessions for six weeks, plus two bimonthly booster sessions. Parents receiving the intervention learned to become aware of emotions in themselves and their children, to acknowledge, label, and empathize with their children's feelings, to engage in problem solving, and to apply regulation strategies for more intense emotions. Parents and children in both groups were assessed before and after the first group received the intervention, and again 6 months later. Compared to the control group, parents in the intervention group became more aware of emotions and engaged in more emotion coaching, and their children showed greater gains in emotion knowledge and greater reductions in the number of behavior problems reported by their teachers and parents.[64] The results suggest that children benefit psychologically when their parents provide guidance in emotion management, and that it is possible to increase parents' capacity to do this through intervention.

PARENTAL MENTAL HEALTH

As noted earlier, research reveals that parental mental health status significantly predicts children's emotional and behavioral problems. Although much attention in this area has focused on maternal mental health, and depression in particular, meta-analytic results indicate that a variety of mental health difficulties in fathers as well as mothers are associated with both internalizing and externalizing symptoms in children. These effects are relatively small, and findings vary according to the informant, the age of the child, and the nature of the parent's disorder, but research demonstrates a consistent association between psychopathology in parents and children.[65] Interpreting these findings can be challenging, as it is difficult to disentangle the causal pathways that may explain the association between parent and child psychiatric functioning. Parental mental health may influence children through genetic transmission, through effects of psychopathology on the prenatal environment (in the case of maternal mental health), or through effects of mental health on parent behavior. It is also possible that children's emotional and behavioral difficulties cause increases in parental dysfunction, or that environmental stressors such as financial hardship or family conflict cause or exacerbate mental health symptoms in parents and children simultaneously.[66]

Regardless of which causal pathways best explain the association between parental psychopathology and children's maladjustment, it is clear that parents who are struggling with mental health problems of their own have additional challenges to confront in raising their children. Fortunately, recent evidence suggests that such parents may be able to help their children by obtaining help for themselves. For example, one study followed 226 families with one parent receiving evidence-based treatment for depression, as well as 97 low-risk families without depressed parents. The researchers examined the effects of parent symptom remission on 7- to 17-year-old children's functioning over a two-year period. Although children with depressed parents exhibited more difficulties than children with nondepressed parents in general, those whose parents experienced remission of depressive symptoms during the course of the study showed improvements in social and academic functioning and perceived competence, relative to those whose parents remained depressed. Changes in parents' symptoms also predicted changes in depressive symptoms among children, and this association was mediated by parental acceptance. That is, as parents became less depressed they became more accepting of their children, and this in turn led to reductions in child symptoms.[67] These results suggest that depressed parents may be able to improve their children's developmental trajectories by taking steps to address their own mental health needs.

Since depression is a cyclical condition, even when depressed parents receive effective treatment, their families may require additional support. To address this need, a group of psychologists recently developed *Keeping Families Strong*, an intervention for families affected by maternal depression. The program is designed to reduce risks (e.g., inadequate understanding of depression, reduced warmth and communication, compromised parenting behaviors with respect to discipline practices, high stress and family conflict, and low social support) and promote resilience (e.g., supportive parenting, positive family interactions, increased coping skills and feelings of safety and security, and family discussions about depression), among older children and adolescents with depressed mothers. Clinicians deliver the treatment in a multifamily group treatment format, in which children meet in one group while their parents (both depressed and unaffected) meet together in a separate group. During 10 weekly sessions and two monthly booster sessions, clinicians provide participants with information about depression and other difficult emotions, and teach them relevant skills related to parenting, coping, and family communication.[68] Although this intervention has yet to be evaluated experimentally, results of a recent posttreatment follow-up were quite promising, revealing improvements in parent functioning, social support, and family interactions, as well as reductions in children's emotional and behavioral problems.[69]

IMPROVING CHILD OUTCOMES FOLLOWING DIVORCE

About 45 percent of marriages in the United States end in divorce, and half of these involve children. This leaves one-fourth of American children in single-parent homes at any given time—the highest rate in the industrialized world.[70] Compared with children of continuously married parents, children of divorce display poorer academic achievement, self-esteem, and social competence and a higher incidence of school dropout and emotional and behavior problems, including de-pression, antisocial behavior, early sexual activity, adolescent parent-hood, and divorce in their adult lives.[71] Moreover, three independently conducted meta-analyses found that the adjustment problems of chil-dren of divorce have intensified in recent years.[72] Although this picture seems bleak, the good news is that there is much that divorced parents can do to improve their children's outcomes. Children's adjustment difficulties in the aftermath of divorce diminish with improved family functioning, and effective interventions exist that can help divorced parents cope with their own stress and support their children through this difficult transition.

In one impressive intervention experiment addressing the impact of parent training on negative parenting behaviors and outcomes associated with divorce, nearly 150 recently separated mothers of first- to third-grade sons were randomly assigned, two-thirds to an experi-mental group and one-third to a no-intervention control group.[73] The experimental group experienced a 14- 16-session program, one session per week, supplemented by midweek phone calls from the researchers to encourage use of the procedures and to troubleshoot problems. The intervention consisted of intensive teaching of parenting principles, videotapes depicting families using effecting parenting techniques to help their children adjust to the divorce transition, and role-play prac-tice. Mothers also received training in managing their own emotions and in ways to deal with family conflict, including ex-spouses, under the assumption that a parent who could better handle the stresses of her own life would be more likely to implement good parenting prac-tices. Laboratory observations of mother-son interactions, gathered just before the intervention and at 6- and 12-month follow-ups, were used to assess program effects.

Findings revealed that experimental-group mothers reduced their use of coercive parenting over time, whereas control-group mothers became increasingly coercive. In addition, experimental-group moth-ers showed less decay in positive parenting during the transition to a single-parent household. Finally, increases in an overall index of effec-tive parenting predicted improved child adjustment, as rated by par-ents, teachers, and children themselves.

Another similar study, which included 240 families of divorce with a 9- to 12-year-old, demonstrated long-term benefits of a brief but in-tensive parent training program.[74] Children whose mothers attended an 11-week parenting skills class not only showed better immediate adjustment but were functioning more favorably at a six-year follow-up than youths whose parents had not attended the parenting class. In sum, these studies demonstrate that it is possible to prevent many of the deleterious effects of divorce on child development, and that parents have a major role to play in these efforts.

SEEING THE GLASS AS HALF FULL

Parents do not cause all children's mental health problems, nor can they solve them all. (any more than psychotropic medications, psychotherapy, or winning the lottery can). Indeed, as research on interactions among risk and protective factors makes clear, it is important to think about solutions to children's mental health problems incrementally, instead of adopting an all-or-none view about health and illness. Virtually every child experiences a mix of developmental advantages and challenges, and neither parents nor children are perfect.

Parents cannot control their children's genetic makeup or temperamental characteristics. But all parents—including those with genetically or temperamentally vulnerable children—do influence developmental trajectories. Authoritative parents who use proactive and nonphysical discipline techniques, apply emotion coaching strategies to promote emotion regulation, and facilitate and monitor their children's peer relationships, can confer substantial developmental benefits upon their children. Likewise, parents who experience difficulties of their own, either in the form of mental health or marital problems, can take comfort in the knowledge that effective professional help is likely to benefit their children as well as themselves.

Importantly, evidence suggests that children who are at risk for maladaptive development, due to biological factors such as genetic predispositions or environmental circumstances such as family conflict or divorce, may gain even more from the parenting efforts just described than children without these risks. This means that all parents have reasons to approach their caregiving endeavors with a sense of purpose and hope. Instead of dwelling on the past, or focusing on risks and obstacles, we encourage parents to focus their attention and efforts on effective child-rearing strategies they can implement in the present and future to optimize their children's well-being, whatever the mixture of biological predispositions, early experiences, and life conditions that may characterize the current developmental context. Doing so requires an optimistic perspective, in which parents view the glass as half full instead of half empty when assessing their children's strengths, challenges, and potential, and when evaluating their own ability to make a difference in their children's lives. Fortunately, the research evidence supports this positive outlook.

10

Building Healthy Minds: It Takes a Village

Stuart Shanker

Over the past decade, there has been an explosion in the number of children identified with mental health and behavioral problems. Current estimates suggest that as many as half of all children enter kindergarten with self-control issues that are likely to impair their ability to function productively in school. One in five children between the ages of 12 and 17 are said to have a diagnosable mental health problem; and one in six children, a developmental disorder. It is far from clear whether these statistics reflect an increase in incidence rates, a heightened awareness of these problems, a shift in diagnostic criteria, advances in sampling techniques, or all of the above. What is clear, however, is that these numbers represent a massive societal problem, requiring a concerted societal response. But this has not yet happened; instead, we have sought to respond to the problem with our existing medical resources, and the trends there are as worrying as the data reported above.

This paper was inspired by the life's work of Stanley Greenspan and is dedicated to his memory. This research was made possible by the generous support of the Harris Steel Foundation and the Harris family, which made it possible to create the Milton and Ethel Harris Research Initiative. We are also grateful for the support we have received from the Unicorn Foundation, Cure Autism Now, the Public Health Agency of Canada, the Templeton Foundation, and York University. I am deeply indebted to Sharna Olfman for the many helpful comments she made on earlier drafts of this text.

Prescription rates of atypical antipsychotics for middle-class children have doubled over the past decade and quadrupled for children from lower-income families. Antipsychotics, as Sparks and Duncan point out in chapter 5, have become a first-line treatment for an alarming number of vulnerable children and adolescents.[1] Overwhelmed pediatricians with little or no training in developmental psychology and psychiatry are increasingly expected to care for these children as health insurance companies restrict access to specialists. Lacking the time and the training to deal with children who cannot control their anger, pay attention, or have trouble falling asleep, they frequently resort to drug therapies that they may know little about, beyond what they have learned from a pharmaceutical rep. The strain on the family is palpable, while the situation at school is becoming intolerable.

Even more disturbing is the knowledge that the most frequently prescribed drugs, stimulants and antipsychotics, do little to address the underlying causes of the child's difficulties. But what is the alternative: a massive investment in secondary care for children? That would be akin to responding to the medical crisis created by smoking by simply increasing the number of oncologists. Rather, we need to try to address these problems at their source, to embrace a preventative approach to mental health and behavior problems.

One of the reasons that drug therapies for mental health issues intensified in the 1990s was because of the increasingly popular belief that they result from genetically caused neurochemical deficits that could be artificially corrected. There has been a significant advance over the past decade, however, in our knowledge about the developmental origins of these problems, and correspondingly, a growing realization that drugs at best only serve to treat the resulting symptoms. If we want to adopt a preventative approach to mental health and behavior problems, we need to train health professionals and caregivers to support parents' efforts to respond sensitively to their children's needs before psychological disturbances arise or become entrenched.

IN SEARCH OF THE SOURCE

Sociologists and psychologists have recently identified a cluster of individual traits that revolve around poor self-control and are correlated with mental health and behavioral problems. These traits include difficulty delaying gratification and ignoring distractions, poor ability to modulate intense negative emotions, and a higher than average frequency in the number of intense negative emotions that are experienced.[2] This cluster of traits can start to emerge as early as the second year of life.[3]

It must be emphasized, however, that children who exhibit these traits as infants or toddlers are *not* emotionally disturbed. Rather, they might be wired in ways that make them more reactive to stressors, and/or their lives may be replete with more stress than they can deal with. Identifying these children and training caregivers to react more sensitively to their developmental needs can circumvent their greater vulnerability to mental illness or behavior problems later in life.

An important longitudinal study just published by psychologist Terrie Moffit at Duke University confirmed that 4-year-old children who perform poorly on self-control tasks are at a much greater risk of developing mental health and behavioral problems later in life.[4] This kind of research has led the Ministry of Children and Youth Services in the Province of Ontario to introduce a universal screening initiative for 18-month-old infants. Parents can complete a checklist, such as the Nipissing District Developmental Screen, which provides a snapshot of a child's development and a starting-point for discussing their child's needs with their primary care physician. In addition, parents are provided with free tools to help them understand and enhance their child's development. Unlike so many screening programs in the United States, which are heavily funded by the pharmaceutical industry and focus on diagnosis, the emphasis in this government-directed program is on ensuring that parents have the guidance and support they need to ensure that their children's developmental trajectories remain on track and that "states do not become traits."

The cluster of traits that I am referring to here must not be confused with impulsivity. After all, as anyone who has lived through the terrible twos will tell you, *all* toddlers struggle with impulse control. But a small percentage of children have greater than average difficulty learning *how* to control their impulses and emotions, and the critical question we are faced with is how we can best assist these children and their families.

There has been no end of child-rearing authorities over the years who have insisted that toddlers' impulsivity is proof positive that we must not "spare the rod" lest we "spoil the child." Some so-called childhood experts even counsel parents not to indulge a crying infant or to shame a two-year-old when he cannot inhibit his impulses. But research suggests that the opposite is the case. Ignoring a baby's signals, or worse still, punishing a baby who is already in distress, places an already vulnerable child at a higher risk for developing psychological and behavioral problems later in life. Toddlers such as these, who are already in a chronically overstressed state, will quickly become overwhelmed when confronted with developmentally inappropriate forms of punishment. The issue with these toddlers is not they have not been sufficiently disciplined, but rather, that they are not capable of coping with stressors in an effective or efficient manner.

So what is a parent with a distressed or distressing child to do? What is a society to do? Should we resign ourselves to the fact that a certain percentage of children are born with unusually strong impulses that are very difficult to inhibit? Or that some children are born with a faulty braking mechanism that is difficult to repair? Or that some children simply don't want to submit to their parents' wishes? The answer to all of these questions is no.

At this juncture, I need to introduce a subtle but critical distinction between *self-control* and *self-regulation* which is the biological substrate for self-control.[5] A toddler may indeed be growing up in a permissive or authoritarian household that undermines his capacity for self-control, either because he fails to develop the mindfulness or the competencies that underpin self-control, or because his parents are actually exacerbating his stress levels. In other cases, while a toddler may *appear* to lack the discipline or the will to control his behavior, in fact, his autonomic nervous system is in such a depleted state—resulting from a bombardment of stressors that he cannot cope with—that he is subject to sudden and urgent needs and experiences intense frustration and anger if these needs are not instantly met. Such a child might not understand the feelings he is experiencing, or he might not be capable of experiencing different emotional gradations of being mildly annoyed, irritated, angry, and furious. For him, frustration results in a 0–60 reaction: a sudden and overwhelming rage. Unfortunately, his resulting tantrum is a coping mechanism that makes matters considerably worse; for now, on top of all of the biological and social stressors, he has to cope with the physiologically debilitating effects of negative emotions, which are dramatically intensified by the negative emotions that his behavior arouses in others.

PARENTS ARE TO BLAME

While it may seem intuitive that bad behavior results from bad parenting, the actual situation is far more complex because children in contemporary society are dealing with so many stressors that were far less prevalent in past generations, as Sharna Olfman discusses at greater length in chapter 3. While a child might be able to cope with one or two stressors for a brief period of time, exposure to multiple stressors over an extended period of time overwhelms a young child's capacity to cope, especially if his ability to tolerate stress is already compromised. Some of the stressors that are now part of the cultural fabric include the following:

- exposure to neurotoxicants and endocrine disruptors in utero and early childhood (such as mercury, lead, pesticides, and pthalates)
- in utero exposure to alcohol, cigarettes, and drugs (which disrupt the neurosystems that subserve self-regulation)[6]
- in utero exposure to excessive maternal stress[7]
- loss of stability of family life
- declining availability of extended family systems
- decline of stable neighborhoods and communities
- loss of opportunities for parents and children to interact meaningfully such as the family dinner hour[8]
- the loss of opportunity for unstructured creative play[9]
- overexposure to TV, video games, and other forms of artificial stimuli
- limited contact with nature[10]
- limited exercise[11]
- sleep deficits[12]
- fast-food and junk-food diets
- developmentally inappropriate educational stimulation
- overly programmed days that stress parents and children alike

It is precisely because of the complex web of factors outlined above that we are faced with a massive societal problem requiring a concerted societal response. However, when faced with so many daunting issues, it is tempting to point a finger at the parents and charge them with being too lenient toward their wild child. Unfortunately, such a narrow view is deeply entrenched in Western attitudes toward child-rearing,[13] resulting in even greater stress for both parent and child.

With the caveat that good parenting matters a great deal, it is important to recognize that when *responsible* parents are wrongfully blamed for their children's out-of-control behavior, and then coerced or shamed into punishing them, the family gets locked into a vicious cycle. The children become increasingly distressed and distressing, and the parents feel increasingly helpless and ineffectual. It may then feel like the key to the magic kingdom when a physician tells them that their children have a disease that can be corrected with drugs, despite their own misgivings about the effects that these drugs might have on their children's emotional vibrancy and their concerns about metabolic side effects.

A proper study of the origins of the parental responsibility outlook would take us back to Proverbs 23:13–14. These sentiments were echoed in the Victorian era and in the writings of Freud and the founders of behaviorism. In the 1960s, a number of studies were published that reiterated the sentiment that a child's impulsivity is due to lax parenting in the early years of life. It was around this time that Walter Mischel began his groundbreaking research on self-control, in which he showed that a young child's inability to restrain herself in an experimental paradigm designed to provoke anxiety in the face of temptation is a significant predictor of the child's educational outlook and long-term well-being.[14]

At the same time that Mischel was studying the significance of a child's ability to delay gratification, Diana Baumrind was developing her parenting style taxonomy. What Baumrind identified as permissive parenting—the warm but overly indulgent parent who makes few demands on the child and readily gives in to the child's impulses—is associated with poor impulse control and increased aggression in children.[15] Authoritarian parenting—the cold and rejecting parent who makes many demands and uses coercive measures to control the child's behavior—is linked to an increased incidence of mood disorders and behavioral problems in preschoolers.[16] Best of all is authoritative parenting—warm, responsive, and attentive care that is sensitive to a child's needs as Meyers and Berk describe in chapter 9. The most damaging form of parenting is harsh or uninvolved parenting, which is a significant predictor of problems of aggression in an older child.[17]

Baumrind's research resonates with the work of renowned child psychoanalyst Margaret Mahler, who posited that as an infant starts to become more aware of his own wishes and desires, he becomes increasingly engaged in a battle of wills with his mother and frequently resorts to tantrums in order to get his way.[18] She argued that how a mother responds to these challenging behaviors plays a critical role in how well the infant will begin to develop inhibitory control. She believed that it was particularly worrying when a mother responds with anger herself, which can intensify the infant's feelings of anger or helplessness, or when she responds by simply giving in, which fails to help the infant develop inhibitory control.

However, some parents discover that their toddlers are particularly susceptible to tantrums, or take a very long time to calm down once a tantrum begins even when they practice authoritative parenting. These children might be higher in the cluster of traits that I referred to earlier either because of their innate temperaments and/or exposure to the myriad chronic stressors—ubiquitous in Western culture—that overwhelm their coping mechanisms. As a consequence, they may be more reactive to stress than the average child, demonstrate an extreme reaction to restraint, have low frustration tolerance, be high in novelty seeking, demonstrate low harm avoidance, or have low reward dependence.[19] Consequently they may overwhelm their parents' ability to cope.

In the early 1990s, the view emerged that each of the traits described above can be tied to a deficit in the amount of serotonin, dopamine, or noradrenaline that the child produces, or the speed at which she can replace these depleted resources.[20] A child with a neurochemical imbalance was thought to be much more prone to anger or anxiety, and just correcting this deficit by providing a pharmaceutical tune-up would bring about a positive change in the child's behavior.

The reality has turned out to be far different. But at the same time that we were embarking on this pharmaceutical experiment—without realizing that it was an experiment—another group of researchers was charting a very different course in their efforts to understand and respond to these children's behavioral challenges. There is a growing realization that children with a propensity to sudden and intense feelings of frustration, anger, or anxiety can, with sensitive caregiving, learn how to modulate their negative emotions and thereby become much less prone to impulsivity. But what exactly is *sensitive caregiving*, and how can we encourage parents to become more keenly attuned to their children's needs while navigating their way through a cultural minefield that seems to be challenging their child's well-being from a multitude of directions?

GREENSPAN'S THEORY

Stanley Greenspan introduced a new dimension of critical importance to understanding children who are mired in and overwhelmed by negative emotions. On the basis of his clinical observations, he agreed with Mahler that an 18- to 24-month-old toddler is undergoing a psychological transition that lays the foundation for the acquisition of self-control. However, Greenspan believed that the Freudian prescription that a child's infantile rages should be met by a firm response intended to develop an internal "braking mechanism of shame, which leads to inhibition and 'drive restraint'" was too limited.[21] Instead of viewing this important developmental transition in terms of acquiring the (shame induced) desire to restrain her impulses, he explained it in terms of the infant's burgeoning ability to use gestures and language to express her emotions and modulate her desires, with the support of an empathic caregiver.[22]

The young child's emerging capacity to communicate with and understand his caregivers changes the very manner in which he copes with situations that he previously found to be overwhelming. Just knowing that he has tools that can help him to stay calm alters his sense of self-efficacy and his belief in his ability to deal with potentially overwhelming situations.[23] However, more is involved here than language as a regulating mechanism. The key here lies in Greenspan's argument that while there is a close link between self-regulation and self-control they are not one and the same; rather, the latter is made possible by the former. A child must be calmly focused and alert in order to learn the various skills—communicative, self-soothing, anticipatory—that underpin self-control. A child may have the desire and may even have mastered strategies for modulating his anger or anxiety, but his state of arousal has a huge bearing on whether or not he can do so. This is true even before a child begins to develop such a desire.

For example, an infant quickly becomes enraged if her arms are held to her sides.[24] If, however, the baby is hypoaroused at the time, there is generally a muted reaction; and the more the baby is hyperaroused, the more intense is her reaction.[25] To be sure, for biological and possibly genetic reasons, some children seem to be much more susceptible to sudden and overpowering feelings of frustration and anger.[26] But Greenspan argued that even with these children, their development of self-control skills can be significantly enhanced; but to do that, we *first have to work on their self-regulation.*[27]

The heart of the theory that we spelled out in our book *The First Idea* is that it is by being regulated that a child develops the ability to self-regulate.[28] The reason why there is such a close relationship between arousal and impulsivity is both biological and social. Take the biological first: when we are confronted by stressful situations our bodies undergo a number of changes that help us to cope. This set of responses is known as the *fight, flight or freeze* response. For example, blood pressure increases, which in turn increases blood flow to the brain, the sweat glands open to prepare for a cooling response (resulting in the galvanic itches or emotional impulses that we all experience under stress) and various metabolic systems work harder, resulting in urgent demands for a high energy activity, and frustration if an outlet is not provided.[29]

If a child is chronically hypo—or hyperaroused—he has less capacity to *coregulate,* in other words to be responsive to his caregivers' efforts to calm and soothe him if he is angry or agitated, or alternatively to stimulate and energize him if he is sad or despondent. Because it is harder for his parents to up- or down-regulate his emotions, he has less capacity to learn how to self-regulate. A chronically hypo- or hyperaroused child is, by definition, less aware of and responsive to signals (both his own bodily signals and other people's communications), and less able to regulate his facial muscles to give a big smile or an angry glare. He is less able to look where he wants to or away from something that is aversive. His field of awareness is inner directed and dominated by all-consuming negative sensations.

In the first year of life, much of the caregiver's regulating behavior is primarily *proximal,* through touch[30] along with modulating vocalizations and looks. But with an actively mobile toddler, the caregiver must increasingly resort to *distal* modes of emotional signaling (e.g., using voice, gestures, facial expressions, looks) in order to up-or down-regulate her baby as necessary. At around 18 months, the toddler is starting to take a more active role in this process, using emotional signals herself in place of discharge behaviors (such as bursting into loud sobs) in order to communicate her desires or needs. While at a younger age, the child primarily communicated her anger or frustration with a rage response, she now uses emotionally expressive gestures and language to convey her feelings. While developing communicative skills, the child learns how to tame catastrophic feelings like fear and rage, and how to modulate and regulate her behavior and moods.

For example, if the child is annoyed, she can make a look of annoyance or utter an expressive sound or hand gesture. Her mother may respond with a gesture indicating, "I understand," or "OK, I'll get the food more quickly," or indicating "Can't you wait just one more minute?" Her anger may be reduced by the mere awareness that her mother is going to do something, even if she can't do it immediately. Just the sound of her voice signals that she is getting the milk bottle ready and it's coming soon. An even better response is if she uses a soothing voice and meets her at her fast-paced, frantic rhythm of back-and-forth cueing and gradually slows down and calms her by introducing a calming interactional rhythm (i.e., down-regulates her).

Through daily coregulated emotional signaling, the child acquires the capacity to interpret and express increasingly fine-tuned emotions rather than being limited to global or extreme feelings such as rage. The child no longer has to have an all-out tantrum to register his annoyance: he can now convey his displeasure with just a withering look. If mother doesn't agree with him or can't bring that food right away, he can now understand her words or gestures, and they help him to modulate his feelings. If he does escalate up to a tantrum because mother hasn't responded with sufficient speed or empathy, it is after he has communicated his feelings more subtly, not from 0 to 60 in a split second. All of his feelings, ranging from joy and happiness to anger, assertiveness, and sadness are becoming fine-tuned regulated emotional interactions rather than all-or-nothing ones.

THE TRANSITION FROM BEING REGULATED TO SELF-REGULATING

As we explained in our book *The First Idea*, the 18-month-old is beginning to make the critical transition from *being regulated* to *self-regulating* as her capacity to convey her own emotions to others and to understand her caregivers' emotional signals grows. The caregiver's role in this transition remains paramount. The examples above all involve invitations or demands from the child for the caregiver to help him cope with a stressor. But if a caregiver responds to a toddler's emotional intensity with emotional intensity of her own, rather than with soothing and calming gestures, the toddler might become even more anxious. Equally serious is if a caregiver tunes out or freezes in response to a toddler's fear or anxiety.

Of all the infant emotions caregivers have to regulate, perhaps the most difficult is anger, which often begets anger or frustration in themselves, or causes them to shut down or shift attention especially when they can't discern the cause of the child's anger, or the child has trouble picking up or understanding his emotional cues. When a toddler expresses anger that is not regulated by a pattern of back-and-forth signaling and negotiation, but instead is routinely dealt with by caregiver withdrawal, avoidance, or anger, this places the toddler at risk for becoming a child whose dominant emotional state is aggression and impulsivity.

Research strongly suggests that children are biologically predisposed to transition from needing their parents to coregulate their emotions to self-regulating. Thirty years ago, Charles Wenar noted that it takes far more energy for an infant or toddler to have a full blown tantrum than to emphatically say *no*.[31] Tantrums are perhaps the most physiologically taxing mode of behavior a child can adopt, which is one reason why excessive anger has such long-term negative consequences for a child's well-being.[32] But an emotionally overwhelmed baby isn't *choosing* to have a tantrum; the overwhelmed baby isn't capable of choosing anything (which is another way of saying that he is overcome by impulses).

The connections between emotion-regulation and energy-modulation are intricate. An organism is wired to maintain positive emotions (e.g., interest, curiosity), which promote energy. In contrast, negative emotions (e.g., fear, anger, anxiety) drain energy. Hence the child is biologically driven to avoid energy-draining negative emotions and maximize energy-promoting positive emotions.[33] This is why a preponderance of negative emotions is such a potent indicator of excessive stress.

Given how draining and devitalizing a tantrum is, very powerful biological needs must be driving a baby who engages in one. By acquiring the communication skills that enable her to forestall this state, she takes a major step forward in her ability to self-regulate. Not only is the 18-month-old learning how to signal her desires and emotions; more fundamentally, she is learning the connection between bodily sensations and emotions and subsequent physical/emotional states, and developing communicative techniques to avoid aversive feelings. But for certain babies it is very hard to make this transition: *not because they lack a sufficiently strong inhibitory muscle,* and not necessarily because a caregiver is incapable of responding consistently to the baby's tantrums. In many cases, the baby's needs may be overpowering, or the infant may have a very low threshold for coping with stress.

This is not to deny the relevance of limit setting on the part of parents as an essential element in self-regulation. One of the reasons why authoritative parenting is associated with such positive child outcomes is because limits are set in a consistent and supportive manner. Parents set limits precisely because they can anticipate the costs to the child's (and one's own!) nervous system that will otherwise result. And they set limits in the hope that the child will eventually come to do so on his own. But the emphasis here is on *self-regulation,* not *suppression.* That is, on down-regulating an overly aroused state and mitigating the intensity of the child's impulses, rather than trying to suppress them, and thereby helping the child to turn his anger or anxiety into a positive source for energizing his actions and spurring him on to overcome a challenge.[34]

BUILDING HEALTHY MINDS

Ten years ago, Greenspan and I started working on a Building Healthy Minds program, based on the book of the same title that he published in 2000.[35] Our idea was to create multidisciplinary teams built around a primary care physician and involving various early childhood specialists. Given that pediatricians or family doctors see infants and children on a regular basis, we felt that they would be ideal to earmark for specialized training in recognizing self-regulation challenges. Diverse specialists such as early childhood educators would then coach parents on the nature of the stressors their child is trying to cope with and how to best reduce the stress load on the child, thereby enhancing his ability to stay calmly focused and alert.

The program came to a sudden halt, not because there wasn't great interest in such a preventative model, but because I received a grant to create the Milton and Ethel Harris Research Initiative (MEHRI), a state-of-the-art developmental and cognitive neuroscience center at York University in Toronto. The ideas that we had for Building Healthy Minds became the basis for MEHRIT, the relational based form of therapy (based on Greenspan and Wieder's Individual Differences/Relationship Based therapy[36]) for children with autism that we have studied at MEHRI over the past seven years.[37] Still, the desire to introduce some form of Building Healthy Minds program for the general public remained very much on our minds.

With that in mind, I received funding from the International Development Research Centre of Canada to take a group of scientists down to Cuba to study their model of preventative medicine. Our findings are summarized in *Maternal Health and Early Childhood Development in Cuba,* a Report presented to the Canadian government by the Canadian Senate Sub-committee on population health.[38]

The reason that I was so interested in the Cuban model was because they have created a system built around what they call polyclinics that is remarkably similar to the model that Dr. Greenspan and I were considering. Polyclinics are local neighborhood health units designed to promote the integration of science, knowledge transfer, parent education and community mobilization, in addition to providing primary health care. These multidisciplinary clinics are built around a primary care physician, and include nurses, community workers, nutritionists, athletic coaches, early educators, and teachers. The focus is strongly on prevention, beginning with prenatal care and with outreach programs designed to ensure regular visits to the clinic, universal screening, and immunization. They serve as a primary site for medical school training and researchers work closely with parents.

The Cubans recognize that, while the array of environmental stressors discussed earlier can severely strain a child's nervous system, sometimes it is the parental or family environment that is the most toxic. But they approach this issue, not with a blame-the-parent mind-set, but with an understanding that parents who are very young and don't have a support network, or parents who were themselves raised in abusive homes, can benefit greatly when exposed to the ideas outlined in this chapter. It turns out that these parents are very grateful for having the opportunity to participate in parenting groups, where a leader gives them a chance to talk about issues like sleep, hygiene, nutrition, dealing with tantrums, discipline, and age-appropriate expectations.

What impressed us most about the Cuban medical system is how focused they are on identifying the potential sources of mental health and behavioral problems as early as possible and then intervening to reduce the downstream consequences of biological and/or social drains on the child's self-regulation. This is very much the focus of the work we do at MEHRI (http://www.mehri.ca). Our findings indicate that the capacity for self-regulation is critical for healthy development and that a successful intervention should be grounded in the following 10 principles:

1. Figure out why a child is chronically hypo- or hyperaroused and what can be done to reduce the stress load on him.
2. Expand the range of stressors with which the child can cope.

3. Enhance the child's ability to communicate his emotional needs.

4. Expand the child's emotional range.

5. Help the child to become mindful of his own arousal states.

6. Help the child to develop strategies for staying calmly focused and alert.

7. Help parents understand their child's behaviors and develop strategies for dealing with potentially dysregulating (emotionally overwhelming) experiences.

8. Help parents understand the importance of activities that promote optimal self-regulation (e.g., exercise, playing outside, increasing creative playtime, improving diet, beneficial sleep routines, interactive family time, etc.).

9. Help parents understand the importance of limiting activities that inhibit optimal self-regulation: taking the TV out of their child's bedroom, reducing or eliminating screen time, reducing developmentally inappropriate formal educational demands, and so forth.

10. Help parents become mindful of their own arousal states and develop their own self-regulating strategies.

In order for primary care physicians to play the central role that I have outlined, they will need to make a major modality shift, away from treating symptoms with psychiatric drugs to addressing the causes. With each and every child the physician should be working to identify the sources of potential downstream problems and discussing strategies with the family for strengthening the child's developmental trajectory. Even with an older child we need to reduce the impetus to reach for the prescription pad and focus instead on ways to reduce the drains on his nervous system and enhance his capacity to deal with stressors.

The sheer number of infants and toddlers struggling with self-regulation issues should alert us to the undue stress that all children are placed under today. This is the reason why we are encouraging pediatricians to offer, during check-ups, general guidelines to *all* parents to reduce stressors such as, no screen time for children under 2 years, in keeping with the American Academy of Pediatrics Guidelines; and more generally, encouraging all parents to make time for creative play and spending time outdoors. Similarly, no infant should for be babysat or put to sleep or breast-fed in front of a TV; no infant should spend time crawling on a yard sprayed with pesticides.

The pediatrician is the ideal person to deliver this information, perhaps with pamphlets that can be handed out and discussed with parents during their first few visits. But we can go even further with this model. My colleague Lori Nichols, the Senior Health Services Resource Nurse at the Children's Aid Society of Toronto, has shown how even the most routine of office procedures can be transformed into a profound learning experience for doctor and parents alike, once viewed through the lens of self-regulation. This starts from the moment that a family enters the waiting room by observing how they deal with the stress of waiting for an appointment in an environment that, despite the omnipresent aquarium, is rarely designed to maximize self-regulation. Then we want to see how the child responds to being poked and prodded by a strange adult or being weighed and measured on a machine that might be unsteady or noisy. An immunization offers the physician a wonderful opportunity to actually feel and hear through her stethoscope how the child responds to a stressful situation and to observe how parents distract and comfort their child. It also offers an opportunity for the physician to help the child become mindful of his own strategies for dealing with stress ("I saw that, even though you were so scared, your whole body began to calm down when I asked you to take a deep breath"). Even something as innocuous as an eye exam offers a wonderful opportunity to observe how well a child complies with a request or responds to a mild stressor, such as not being able to read a line they find difficult.

If the physician suspects that a child has mild problems in sensory regulation or integration, emotion-regulation, or executive functioning, she can begin discussing effective strategies that the parents can employ to help their child. Just having their attention drawn to how anxious their child was and how calm she became when comforted can have a dramatic effect on a parent's awareness of their child's needs and their own parenting tendencies. Regular immunization visits offer the perfect opportunity to monitor the family's progress in dealing with the myriad stressors that have become ubiquitous in contemporary culture.

We also need to tap into existing resource persons in the community who can work with parents on an ongoing basis to enhance their awareness of the often very subtle signs children display that reveal that they are overstressed or to develop strategies for helping their children stay calmly focused and alert. Caregivers and early childhood educators are invaluable. We have found in our work with early childhood educators, who already have a strong background in human development, that they are remarkably effective at implementing individualized programs based on Jean Ayers's ideas about sensory integration and Stanley Greenspan's ideas about enhancing communicative skills. And programs like Kids Have Stress Too! have demonstrated that it is possible to teach even preschoolers strategies for remaining calmly focused and alert, and to provide teachers and parents with practices that enhance such mindfulness.[39]

What about enhancing the child's emotional range? Programs like Roots of Empathy have shown how in-class activities led by instructors trained in social-emotional learning can have a powerful effect on a child's ability to modulate their negative emotions or to understand what others are thinking and feeling.[40] And programs like Tools of Mind have shown that it is possible to teach meta-cognitive strategies while at the same time working on literacy and numeracy.[41]

Coaches, choir leaders, art and drama teachers, mentors, families who go for long nature walks on the weekend, the scouts, the Y, 4-H, and Right to Play: there are no end of potential mentors and activities to promote healthy self-regulation in children. But this isn't just about the beneficial effects of such activities on the autonomic nervous system[42]: it is just as much a story about weaning the child from those sources of a rapid energy fix such as fast food and electronic media, that undermine the child's ability to respond to stressors.

If we are serious about reducing the use of psychiatric drugs to control children's out-of-control emotions and behaviors, then we need a broad-based effort, addressing all of the different elements involved in optimal self-regulation. And the starting-point is to reframe children's behavior for parents, teachers, doctors, and policy makers. We need everyone to understand that there is no such a thing as a bad child, a lazy child, or a dull child. But if we do the wrong things we can certainly cultivate these traits in our children.

We especially need parents to understand that some children are wired to find very elementary actions, like sitting up or walking or going downstairs very taxing; that some children have trouble knowing when they are hungry or tired or cold; that some children become very anxious or excited when they are exposed to bright lights or noisy environments or strong smells or new tastes and textures, or even just to people who gesture a lot or who speak very quickly; that some children find learning itself very taxing, both physiologically and emotionally; or that some children find it very difficult to express what they are feeling. Still other children may be overwhelmed by stressors that are ubiquitous in contemporary culture such as violent media, developmentally inappropriate academic demands, lack of access to the outdoors, exposure to toxins, and so forth.

The better parents understand the reasons why their child might be acting up, or not paying attention, or having trouble falling asleep, or being aggressive on the playground, or insensitive to the feelings of others, the better they can help her to stay regulated. The better the child can stay regulated, the better she will learn how to regulate herself. And the better she can self-regulate, the greater will be her capacity to harness all that energy so that, instead of fueling out-of-control behaviors that we are trying to suppress with drugs, it can be channeled into great works of art and science.

Afterword

Sharna Olfman

The rich diversity of cultures created by humankind is a testament to our ability to develop and adapt in diverse ways. But however varied different cultures may be, children are not endlessly malleable; they all share basic psychological and physical needs that must be met to ensure healthy development. The Childhood in America series examines the extent to which American culture meets children's irreducible needs. Without question, many children growing up in the United States lead privileged lives. They have been spared the ravages of war, poverty, malnourishment, sexism, and racism. However, despite our nation's resources, not all children share these privileges. Additionally, values that are central to American culture, such as self-reliance, individualism, privacy of family life, and consumerism, have created a climate in which parenting has become intolerably labor intensive, and children are being taxed beyond their capacity for healthy adaptation. Record levels of psychiatric disturbance, violence, poverty, apathy, and despair among our children speak to our current cultural crisis.

Although our elected officials profess their commitment to family values, policies that support family life are woefully lacking and inferior to those in other industrialized nations. American families are burdened by inadequate parental leave, a health care system that does not provide universal coverage for children, a minimum wage that is not a living wage, welfare-to-work policies that require parents to leave their children for long stretches of time, unregulated and inadequately subsidized day care, an unregulated entertainment industry that exposes children to sex and violence, and a two-tiered public education system that delivers inferior education to poor children and frequently ignores individual differences in learning styles and profiles of intelligence. As a result, many families are taxed to the breaking point. In addition, our fascination with technological innovation is creating a family lifestyle that is dominated by the screen rather than human interaction.

The Childhood in America series seeks out leading childhood experts from across the disciplines to promote dialogue, research, and understanding regarding how best to raise and educate psychologically healthy children, to ensure that they will acquire the wisdom, heart, and courage needed to make choices for the betterment of society.

Notes

INTRODUCTION

1. Spielmans, G. I., & Parry, P. I. (2010). From Evidence-Based Medicine to Marketing-Based Medicine: Evidence from Internal Industry Documents. *Bioethical Inquiry.* Retrieved from http://i.bnet.com/blogs/spielmans-parry-ebm-to-mbm-jbioethicinqu-2010.pdf; Robbins, B. D., Higgins, M., Fisher, M., & Over, K. (2011). Conflicts of interest in research on antipsychotic treatment of pediatric bipolar disorder, temper dysregulation disorder, and attenuated psychotic symptoms syndrome: Exploring the unholy alliance between big pharma and psychiatry. *Journal of Psychological Issues in Organizational Culture, 1*(4), 32–49.

2. Zito, J. M., & Safer, D. J. (2005). Recent Child Pharmacoepidemiological Findings. *Journal of Child and Adolescent Psychopharmacology, 15*(1), 5–9.

3. Olfson, M., Crystal, S., Huang, C., & Gerhard, T. (2010). Trends in Antipsychotic Drug Use by Very Young, Privately Insured Children. *Journal of the American Academy of Child & Adolescent Psychiatry, 49*(1), 13–23.

4. Crystal, S., Olfson, M., Huang, C., Pincus, H., & Gerhard, T. (2009). Broadened Use of Atypical Antipsychotics; Safety, Effectiveness, & Policy Challenges. *Health Affairs, 28*(5), w770–w781.

5. Gottstein, J. B. (2009, October). *Litigating Against the Psychiatric Drugging of Children & Youth.* ICSPP Annual Conference, Syracuse, NY.

6. Crystal et al., Broadened Use of Atypical Antipsychotics; Duff, W. (2009, December 11). Poor Children Likelier to get Antipsychotics. *New York Times.* Retrieved from http://www.nytimes.com/2009/12/12/health/12medicaid.html?_r=1.

7. Whitaker, R. (2002). *Mad in America.* New York: Basic Books.

8. Waters, R. (2005, May/June). Medicating Aliah. *Mother Jones.*

9. Whitaker, *Mad in America,* p. 277.

10. Ibid., p. 279.

11. Ibid.

12. Ibid., p. 281.

13. Olfson et al., Trends in Antipsychotic Drug Use.

14. Sheller, S. (2009, October). *Keynote Address.* ISPP Annual Conference, Syracuse, NY.

15. Ibid.

16. Olfson et al., Trends in Antipsychotic Drug Use.

17. Healy, D. (2007). Bipolar Syndrome by Proxy? The Case of Pediatric Bipolar Disorder. In Sharna Olfman, Ed., *Bipolar Children: Cutting Edge Controversy, Insight, and Research.* Praeger Press, Westport, CT; Healy, D. (2003). *Let Them Eat Prozac.* Toronto: James Lorimer & Company, pp. 12–13; Whitaker, *Mad in America.*

18. Diller, L. (2007). But Don't Call It Science. In Sharna Olfman, Ed., *Bipolar Children: Cutting Controversy, Insight, and Research* (pp. 28–45). Westport, CT: Praeger Publishers; Harris, G. (2009, March 19). Drug Maker Told Studies Would Aid It, Papers Say. *New York Times.* Retrieved from http://www.nytimes.com/2009/03/22/us/20psych.html; Kowalczyk, L. (2009, March 21). Senator broadens inquiry into psychiatrist. *Boston Globe,* p. B.1, Metro.

19. Whitaker, *Mad in America,* p. 281.

20. Healy, D., & Le Noury, J. (2007). Bipolar Syndrome by Proxy? The Case of Pediatric Bipolar Disorder. In Sharna Olfman, Ed., *Bipolar Children: Cutting Controversy, Insight, and Research, Praeger Publishers.* Westport, CT: Praeger Publishers.

21. Olfson et al., Trends in Antipsychotic Drug Use.

22. Olfman, S. (Ed.). (2006). *No Child Left Different.* Westport, CT: Praeger Publishers.

23. Olfman, S. (Ed.). (2005). *Childhood Lost.* Westport, CT: Praeger Publishers.

24. Carey, B. (2010, February 10). Revising Book on Disorders of the Mind. *New York Times.* Retrieved from http://www.nytimes.com/2010/02/10/health/10psych.html.

CHAPTER 1

1. J. Zito, "Psychotropic practice patterns for youth," *Arch Pediatr Adolesc Med* 157 (2003): 17–25.

2. This number is based upon the prescribing rates cited for the two populations, children under age 18 with private insurance and children covered by Medicaid. I assumed that children who didn't have health insurance were prescribed antipsychotics at the same rate as those covered by health insurance.

3. C. Moreno, "National trends in the outpatient diagnosis and treatment of bipolar disorder in youth," *Arch Gen Psychiatry* 64 (2007): 1032–39.

4. Deposition of Joseph Biederman in legal case of *Avila v. Johnson & Johnson Co.,* Feb. 26, 2009, pp. 139, 231, 232, 237.

5. J. Biederman, "Attention-deficit hyperactivity disorder and juvenile mania," *J Am Acad Child & Adolesc Psychiatry* 35 (1996): 997–1008.

6. Deposition of Joseph Biederman, p. 158.

7. G. Harris, "Researchers fail to reveal full drug pay," *New York Times,* June 8, 2008.

8. Deposition of Joseph Biederman, p. 119.

9. J. Biederman, *Annual Report 2002: The Johnson & Johnson Center for Pediatric Psychopathology at the Massachusetts General Hospital.*

10. C. Moreno, "National trends."

11. R. Waters, "J&J, Pfizer Profit on 'Juvenile Bipolar Juggernaut,'" *Bloomberg News*, Sept. 5, 2007.

12. M. Olfson, "National trends in the outpatient treatment of children and adolescents with antipsychotic drugs," *Arch Gen Psychiatry* 63 (2006): 679–85.

13. B. Vitiello, "Antipsychotics in children and adolescents," *Eur Neuropsychopharmacol* 19 (2009): 629–35; C. Panagiotopoulos, "First do no harm," *J Can Acad Child Adolesc Psychiatry* 19 (2010): 124–37.

14. P. Weiden, *Breakthroughs in Antipsychotic Medications* (New York: W.W. Norton, 1999), p. 26.

15. E. Nestler and S. Hyman, *Molecular Neuropharmacology* (New York: McGraw Hill, 2002), p. 392.

16. H. Nasrallah, "Atypical antipsychotic-induced metabolic side effects," *Mol Psychiatry* 13 (2008): 27–35.

17. Ibid. Also see M. DeHert, "Metabolic and endocrine adverse effects of second-generation antipsychotics in children and adolescents," *Eur Psychiatry* (2011), doi:10.1016.

18. C. Correll, "Antipsychotic use in children and adolescents," *J Am Acad Child Adolesc Psychiatry* 47 (2008): 9–20.

19. DeHert, "Metabolic and endocrine adverse effects"; Nasrallah, "Atypical antipsychotic-induced metabolic side effects."

20. D. Fraguas, "Efficacy and safety of second-generation antipsychotics in children and adolescents with psychotic and bipolar spectrum disorders," *Eur Neuropsychopharmacol* (2010), doi:10.1016.

21. L. Sikich, "Double-blind comparison of first-and second-generation antipsychotics in early-onset schizophrenia and schizoaffective disorder," *Am J Psychiatry* 165 (2008): 1420–31.

22. Vitiello, "Antipsychotics in children and adolescents."

23. DeHert, "Metabolic and endocrine adverse effects."

24. Vitiello, "Antipsychotics in children and adolescents."

25. Panagiotopoulos, "First do no harm."

26. R. Findling, "Double-blind maintenance safety and effectiveness findings from the treatment of early-onset schizophrenia spectrum (TEOSS) study," *J Am Acad Child & Adolesc Psychiatry* 49 (2010): 583–94.

27. NIMH press release, May 17, 2010, "Effectiveness of long-term use of antipsychotic medication to treat childhood schizophrenia is limited."

28. L. Sikich, "A pilot study of risperidone, olanzapine, and haloperidol in psychotic youth," *Neuropsychopharmacology* 29 (2004): 133–45.

29. Correll, "Antipsychotic use in children and adolescents."

30. Ibid. Also, C. Correll, "Assessing and maximizing the safety and tolerability of antipsychotics used in the treatment of children and adolescents," *J Clin Psychiatry* 69, suppl. 4 (2008): 26–36.

31. I. Wonodi, "Tardive dyskinesia in children treated with atypical antipsychotic medications," *Mov Disord* 22 (2007): 1777–82.

32. P. Laita, "Antipsychotic-related abnormal involuntary movements and metabolic and endocrine side effects in children and adolescents," *J Child Adolesc Psychopharmacol* 17 (2007): 487–502.

33. C. Arango, "Olanzapine compared to quetiapine in adolescents with a first psychotic episode," *Eur Child & Adolesc Psychiatry* 18 (2009): 418–28.

34. G. Ratzoni, "Weight gain associated with olanzapine and risperidone in adolescent patients," *J Am Acad Child Adolesc Psychiatry* 41 (2002): 337–43.

35. C. Pangiotopoulos, "Increased prevalence of obesity and glucose intolerance in youth treated with second-generation antipsychotic medications," *Can J Psychiatry* 54 (2009): 743–49; N. Patel. "Body mass indexes and lipid profiles in hospitalized children and adolescents exposed to atypical antipsychotics," *J Child & Adolesc Psychopharmacol* 17 (2007): 303–11.

36. Fraguas, "Efficacy and safety of second-generation antipsychotics"; DeHert, "Metabolic and endocrine adverse effects."

37. Panagiotopoulos, "First do no harm."

38. Ibid.

39. Patel, "Body mass indexes and lipid profiles."

40. Panagiotopoulos, "First do no harm."

41. Vitiello, "Antipsychotics in children and adolescents."

42. Laita, "Antipsychotic-related abnormal involuntary movements."

43. See DeHert, "Metabolic and endocrine adverse effects"; Vitiello, "Antipsychotics in children and adolescents"; Laita, "Antipsychotic-related abnormal involuntary movements"; Panagiotopoulos, "First do no harm"; and C. Correll, "Endocrine and metabolic adverse effects of psychotropic medications in children and adolescents," *J Acad Child Adolesc Psychiatry Am* 45 (2006): 771–90.

44. See De Hert, "Metabolic and endocrine adverse effects"; Panagiotopoulos, "First do no harm."

45. R. McIntyre, "Metabolic and cardiovascular adverse events associated with antipsychotic treatment in children and adolescents," *Arch Pediatr Adolesc Med* 162 (2008): 929–35. Also see De Hert, "Metabolic and endocrine adverse effects"; Panagiotopoulos, "First do no harm."

46. See Laita, "Antipsychotic-related abnormal involuntary movements"; De Hert, "Metabolic and endocrine adverse effects."

47. Correll, "Antipsychotic use in children and adolescents." Also see De Hert, "Metabolic and endocrine adverse effects."

48. Findling, "Double-blind maintenance safety and effectiveness findings."

49. Ibid.

50. L. Sikich, "Double-blind comparison of first-and second-generation antipsychotics." Also see Correll, "Assessing and maximizing the safety and tolerability of antipsychotics"; J. Jerrell, "Neurological adverse events associated with antipsychotic treatment in children and adolescents," *J Child Neurol* 23 (2008): 1392–99.

51. Findling, "Double-blind maintenance safety and effectiveness findings."

52. J. Jerrell, "Adverse events in children and adolescents treated with antipsychotic medications," *Hum Psychopharmacol* 23 (2008): 283–90.

53. J. Wade, "Tardive dyskinesia and cognitive impairment," *Biol Psychiatry* 22 (1987): 393–95.

54. M. Myslobodsky, "Central determinants of attention and mood disorder in tardive dyskinesia," *Brain Cognition* 23 (1993): 56–70.

55. B. Ho, "Progressive structural brain abnormalities and their relationship to clinical outcome," *Arch Gen Psychiatry* 60 (2003): 585–94. N; Andreasen, "Longitudinal changes in neurocognition during the first decade of schizophrenia illness," *Int Cong Schiz Res* (2005): 348.

56. K. Dorph-Petersen, "The influence of chronic exposure to antipsychotic medications on brain size before and after tissue fixation," *Neuropsychopharmacology* 30 (2005): 1649–61.

57. B. Ho, "Long term antipsychotic treatment and brain volume," *Arch Gen Psychiatry* 68 (2011): 128–37.

58. M. Morgan, "Prospective analysis of premature mortality in schizophrenia in relation to health service engagement," *Psychiatry Res* 117 (2003): 127–35; S. Saha, "A systematic review of mortality in schizophrenia," *Arch Gen Psychiatry* 64 (2007): 1123–31; M. Joukamaa, "Schizophrenia, neuroleptic medication, and mortality," *Br J Psychiatry* 188 (2006): 122–27.

59. C. Colton, "Congruencies in increased mortality rates, years of potential life lost, and causes of death among public mental health clients in eight states," *Prev Chronic Dis* 3 (April 2006).

CHAPTER 2

1. McIntyre, D. A. (2010, May 19). Big pharma makes more money on kids, use of medications among the young rises. 247wallst.com, n.p. Retrieved from http://247wallst.com/2010/05/19/big-pharma-makes-more-money-on-kids-use-of-medications-among-the-young-rises/.

2. Kozel, M. (2011, February 5). Little pharma: The medication of U.S. children. Huffington Post.com, n.p. Retrieved from http://www.huffingtonpost.com/maggie-kozel-md/childrens-health-care_b_803167.html.

3. Olson, J. (2011, June 23). Bipolar label soars among kids. *StarTribune*, n.p. Retrieved from http://www.startribune.com/lifestyle/wellness/124136764.html.

4. Donaldson, L. (2010, May 3). Psychiatric drugging of American children is cause for alarm. *Portland Press Herald*, n.p. http://www.pressherald.com/opinion/psychiatric-drugging-of-american-children-is-cause-for-alarm_2010-05-03.html.

5. Olfson, M., Blanco, C., Liu, L., Moreno, C., & Laje, G. (2006). National trends in the outpatient treatment of children and adolescents with antipsychotic drugs. *Archives of General Psychiatry, 63*(6), 679–685.

6. Szalavitz, M. (2011, May 26). Drugging the vulnerable: Atypical antipsychotics in children and the elderly. *Time*, n.p. Retrieved from http://healthland.time.com/2011/05/26/why-children-and-the-elderly-are-so-drugged-up-on-antipsychotics/print/; Kaplan, A. (2011, May 23). Nearly half of kids in inpatient psychiatric program receive antipsychotics. *Psychiatric Times*, n.p. Retrieved from http://www.psychiatrictimes.com/conference-reports/apa2011/content/article/10168/1865851.

7. Llorente, M. D., & Urrutia, V. (2006). Diabetes, psychiatry disorders, and the metabolic effects of antipsychotic medications. *Clinical Diabetes, 24*(1), 18–24.

8. Barnes, T.R.E., & Braude, W. M. (1985). Akathisia variants and tardive dyskinesia. *Archives of General Psychiatry, 42*(9), 874–878.

9. Ho, B. C., Andreason, N. C., Zieball, S., Pierson, R., & Magnota, V. (2011). Long-term antipsychotic treatment and brain volume: A longitudinal study of first-episode schizophrenia. *Archives of General Psychiatry, 28*(2), 128–137.

10. Whitaker, R. (2010). *Anatomy of an epidemic: Magic bullets, psychiatry drugs, and the astonishing rise of mental illness in America.* New York: Crown Publishers.

11. Herper, M. (2004, Sept.). Antipsychotic prescribed as sleeping pill. Forbes. com, n.p. Retrieved from http://www.forbes.com/2004/09/08/cx_mh_0908sero quel.html.

12. Donaldson, Psychiatric drugging of American children.

13. Wilson, D. (2010, Sept. 1). Child's ordeal shows risks of psychosis drugs for the young. *New York Times,* n.p. Retrieved from http://www.nytimes.com/ 2010/09/02/business/02kids.html?pagewanted=all.

14. Olson, Bipolar label soars among kids.

15. Donaldson, Psychiatric drugging of American children.

16. Rushton, J. L., Clark, S. J., & Freed, G. L. (2000). Pediatrician and family physician prescription of selective serotonin reuptake inhibitors. *Pediatrics, 105*(6), e82.

17. AAP Department of Community and Specialty Pediatrics. (2010, July). Resources help primary care clinicians address mental health concerns. *AAP News, 31*(7), 34.

18. Kim, W. J. (2003). Child and adolescent psychiatry workforce: A critical shortage and national challenge. *Academic Psychiatry, 27,* 277–282.

19. Donaldson, Psychiatric drugging of American children.

20. Laforgia, M. (2011, May 24). Huge doses of potent antipsychotics flow into state jails for troubled kids. *Palm Beach Post,* n.p. http://www.psychsearch.net/ psych_news/?p=1697.

21. Ibid.

22. Zito, J. M., Safer, D. J., Sai, D., Gardener, J. F., Thomas, D., Coombes, P., . . . Mendez-Lewis, M. (2008). Psychotropic medication patterns among youth in foster care. *Pediatrics, 121*(1), e157–163.

23. Kaplan, Nearly half of kids in inpatient psychiatric program receive antipsychotics.

24. Donaldson, Psychiatric drugging of American children.

25. Whitaker, R. (2002). *Mad in America: Bad science, bad medicine, and the enduring mistreatment of the mentally ill.* New York: Basic Books.

26. Charland, L. C. (2007). Benevolent theory: Moral treatment at the York retreat. *History of Psychiatry, 18*(1), 61–80.

27. Whitaker, *Mad in America,* p. 27.

28. Whitaker, *Mad in America;* Dowbiggin, I. R. (1997). *Keeping America sane: Psychiatry and eugenics in the United States and Canada 1880–1940.* Ithaca, NY: Cornell University Press; Black, E. (2003). *War against the weak: Eugenics and America's campaign to create a master race.* New York: Four Walls Eight Windows.

29. Whitaker, *Mad in America.*

30. Illich, I. (2000). *Limits to medicine: Medical nemesis, the expropriation of health.* London: Marion Boyars Press.

31. Whitaker, *Mad in America.*

32. Dowbiggin, *Keeping America sane.*

33. Malthus, T. (2008/1798). *An essay on the principle of population.* Oxford: Oxford University Press.

34. Galton, F. (2004). *Essays in eugenics.* Honolulu, HI: University Press of the Pacific.

35. Chung, M. C., & Nolan, P. (1998). Children and challenging behaviour: Past and present in the United Kingdom. *Children and Society, 12,* 251–262.

36. Chung & Nolan, Children and challenging behaviour, p. 252.

37. Whitaker, *Mad in America*, p. 52.

38. Ibid., p. 60.

39. Ibid., p. 63.

40. Kiesler, D. (2000). *Beyond the disease model of mental disorders.* Santa Barbara, CA: Praeger.

41. Felder, A. J., & Robbins, B. D. (2011). A cultural-existential approach to therapy: Merleau-Ponty's phenomenology of embodiment and its implications for practice. *Theory and Psychology, 21*(3).

42. Pescosolido, B. A., Martin, J. K., Long, S., Medina, T. R., Phelan, J. C., & Link, B. G. (2010). "A disease like any other"? A decade of change in public reactions to schizophrenia, depression, and alcohol dependence. *American Journal of Psychiatry, 167,* 1321–1330.

43. Elkins, D. N. (2009). *Humanistic psychology: A clinical manifesto.* Colorado Springs, CO: University of the Rockies Press; Mosher, L. R., & Hendrix, V. (2004). *Soteria: Through madness to deliverance.* Bloomington, IN: Xlibris; Duncan, B. L., Miller, S. D., Wampold, B. E., & Hubble, M. A. (Eds.). (2009). *The heart and soul of change: Delivering what works in therapy* (2nd ed.). Washington, DC: American Psychological Association.

44. Hellerman, C. (2011, July 22). Cocaine: The evolution of the once "wonder" drug. CNN, n.p. Retrieved from http://www.koco.com/r/28638691/detail.html.

45. Ibid.

46. El-Hai, J. (2005). *The lobotomist: A maverick genius and his tragic quest to rid the world of mental illness.* New York: Wiley.

47. LeDoux, J. (1996). The emotional brain. In J. M. Jenkins, K. Oatley, & N. L. Stein (Eds.), *Human emotions: A reader* (pp. 98–111). Malden, MA: Blackwell.

48. Whitaker, *Mad in America.*

49. Ibid.

50. Hunt, M. (1994). *The story of psychology.* Norwell, MA: Anchor.

51. Oh, V.M.S. (1994). The placebo effect: Can we use it better? *British Medical Journal, 309,* 69; Shapiro, A. K. (1964). A historic and heuristic definition of the placebo. *Psychiatry, 27,* 52–80.

52. Patel, S. M., Stason, W. B., Legedza, A., Ock, S. M., Kaptchuk, T. J., Conboy, L., . . . Lembo, A. J. (2005). The placebo effect in irritable bowel syndrome trials: A meta-analysis. *Neurograstroenterology & Motility, 17*(3), 332–340.

53. Kirsch, I. (2010). *The emperor's new drugs: Exploding the antidepressant myth.* New York: Basic Books.

54. Fournier, J., DeRubeis, R., Hollon, S., Dimidjian, S., Amsterdam, J., Shelton, R., & Fawcett, J. (2010). Antidepressant drug effects and depression severity: A patient-level meta-analysis. *JAMA, 303*(1), 47–53.

55. Kirsch, *The emperor's new drugs.*

56. Angell, M. (2011, June 23). The epidemic of mental illness: Why? *New York Review of Books,* n.p.; Angell, M. (2011, July 11). The illusions of psychiatry. *New York Review of Books,* n.p. Retrieved from

57. Kirsch, *The emperor's new drugs*; Whitaker, *Anatomy of an epidemic*; Carlat, D. (2010). *Unhinged: The trouble with psychiatry—a doctor's revelations about a profession in crisis.* New York: Free Press.

58. Faille, C. (2011, July 12). Investing for a backlash against psychopharmacology. *Forbes.*

59. Whitaker, *Anatomy of an epidemic,*.

60. Robbins, B. D., Higgins, M., Fisher, M., & Over, K. (2011). Conflicts of interest in research on antipsychotic treatment of pediatric bipolar disorder, temper dysregulation disorder, and attenuated psychotic symptoms syndrome: Exploring the unholy alliance between big pharma and psychiatry. *Journal of Psychological Issues in Organizational Culture, 1*(4), 32–49.

61. Cosgrove, L., Krimsky, S., Vijayaraghavan, M., & Schneider, L. (2006). Financial ties between DSM-IV panel members and the pharmaceutical industry. *Psychotherapy and Psychosomatics, 75,* 154–160.

62. Cosgrove, L. (2010, April). *Re-thinking the meaning of "evidence-based medicine" in an industry dominated climate.* Keynote address at the Undergraduate Humanities and Human Sciences Conference, Point Park University, Pittsburgh, PA.

63. American Psychiatric Association. (2010a). DSM-5 development: Temper dysregulation disorder with dysphoria. Retrieved from http://www.dsmt.org; American Psychiatric Association. (2010b). Justification for temper dysregulation with dysphoria. Retrieved from http://www.dsm5.org; American Psychiatric Association. (2010c). Attention psychotic symptoms syndrome. Retrieved from http://www.dsm5.org

64. Frances, A. (2010a). DSM-5 temper dysregulation—good intentions, bad solution. *Psychology Today,* n.p.

65. Rusch, N., Corrigan, P. W., Todd, A. R., & Bodenhausen, G. V. (2010). Implicit self-stigma in people with mental illness. *Journal of Nervous Mental Disease, 198,* 150–153.

66. Frances, A. (2010b). DSM-5 "psychosis risk syndrome"—far too risky. *Psychology Today,* n.p.

67. Felder and Robbins, A cultural-existential approach to therapy.

CHAPTER 3

1. U.S. Census Bureau. (2002b). *Statistical abstract of the United States* (123rd ed.). Washington, DC: U.S.

2. Berk, L. E. (2005). Why parenting matters. In Olfman, S. (Ed.) *Childhood lost* (pp. 19–53). Westport, CT: Praeger.

3. Olfman, S. (Ed.). (2005). *Childhood lost.* Westport, CT: Praeger.

4. Cavoukian, R., & Olfman, S. (Eds.). (2006). *Child honoring: How to turn this world around.* Westport, CT: Praeger.

5. Bronfenbrenner, U. (1988). Strengthening family systems. In E. F. Zigler & M. Frank (Eds.), *The parental leave crisis: Toward a national policy* (pp. 143–160). New Haven, CT: Yale University Press.

6. Schore, A. (2003). *Affect dysregulation and disorders of the self.* New York: Norton.

7. Karen, R. (1998). *Becoming attached: First relationships and how they shape our capacity to love.* New York: Oxford University Press.

8. Ibid., p. 3.

9. Small, M. (2004). The natural history of children. In S. Olfman (Ed.), *Childhood lost: How American culture is failing our kids* (pp. 3–18). Westport, CT: Praeger.

10. Ibid.

11. Karen, *Becoming attached,* p. 3. Small, The natural history of children.

12. Stern, D. (1985). *The interpersonal world of the infant.* New York: Basic Books.

13. Rice, R. S. (1997). Neurophysiological development in premature infants following stimulation. *Developmental Psychology, 13,* 69–76; White, J. L., & Labarba, R. C. (1976). The effects of tactile and kinesthetic stimulation on neonatal development in the premature infant. *Developmental Psychobiology, 9,* 569–77.

14. McKenna, J. J., Mosko, S. S., Richard, C., Drummond, S., Hunt, L., Cetel, M. B. & Arpaia, J. (1994). Experimental studies of infant-parent co-sleeping: Mutual physiological and behavioral influences and their relevance to SIDS (sudden infant death syndrome). *Early Human Development, 38,* 187–201.

15. Angier, N. (1994, May 24). Mother's milk found to be potent cocktail of hormones. *New York Times,* p. B5.

16. Gerehardt, S. (2004). *Why love matters: How affection shapes a baby's brain.* New York: Brunner-Routledge.

17. Schore, *Affect dysregulation and disorders of the self.*

18. Gerehardt, *Why love matters.*

19. Ibid.

20. Ibid.

21. Baumrind, D. (1971). Current patterns of parental authority. *Developmental Psychology Monograph, 4*(1, Pt. 2); Kuczynski, L. & Lollis, S. (2002). Four foundations for a dynamic model of parenting. In J.R.M. Gerris (Ed.), *Dynamics of parenting.* Hillsdale, NJ: Erlbaum; Russell, A., Mize J., & Bissaker K. (2002). Parent-child relationships. In P. K. Smith & C. Hart (Eds.), *Handbook of childhood social development.* Oxford, UK: Blackwell.

22. Berk, L. E. (2005). *Infants, children and adolescents.* Boston: Pearson & Allyn and Bacon.

23. Erikson, E. H. (1950). *Childhood and society.* New York: Norton.

24. Harlow, H. F., & Zimmerman, R. (1959). Affectional responses in the infant monkey. *Science, 130,* 421–432; Small, M. F. (1999). *Our babies, ourselves: How biology and culture shape the way we parent.* New York: Anchor Books.

25. Bronfenbrenner, U. (1988). Strengthening family systems. In E. F. Zigler & M. Frank (Eds.), *The parental leave crisis: Toward a national policy* (pp. 143–160). New Haven, CT: Yale University Press.

26. Bronfenbrenner, U. (1992). Child care in the Anglo-Saxon mode. In M. E. Lamb, J. J. Sternberg, C. P. Hwang & A. G. Broberg (Eds.), *Child care in context* (pp. 281–291). Hillsdale, NJ: Lawrence Erlbaum.

27. Berk, *Why parenting matters.*

28. Ibid.

29. Bronfenbrenner, U. (1985). The future of childhood. In V. Greaney (Ed.), *Children: Needs and rights* (pp. 167–186). New York: Irvington Publishers.

CHAPTER 4

1. John Breeding, PhD, and Amy Philo, "Relentless and Tragic Marketing: Psychiatric Drugs from Before the Cradle to the Grave," *Unite for Life,* Nov. 8, 2010, http://uniteforlife.wordpress.com/2010/11/08/relentless-and-tragic-marketing-psychiatric-drugs-from-before-the-cradle-to-the-grave-by-john-breeding-phd-and-amy-philo/.

2. Robert Whitaker, *Anatomy of an Epidemic: Magic Bullets, Psychiatric Drugs, and the Astonishing Rise of Mental Illness in America* (New York: Crown Publishers, 2010), 3.

3. Bill Bekrot, "Prescription Drug Use by US Children on the Rise," Reuters, May 19, 2010, http://www.reuters.com/article/2010/05/19/medco-children-idUSN1924289520100519.

4. Ibid.

5. Dr. Joseph Mercola, "Selling Fear and Sickness," Mercola, Sept. 29, 2005, http://articles.mercola.com/sites/articles/archive/2005/09/29/selling-fear-and-sickness.aspx.

6. Breeding and Philo, "Relentless and Tragic Marketing."

7. Whitaker, *Anatomy of an Epidemic*, 318.

8. Ibid., 319.

9. "Joseph Biederman," *Wikipedia the Free Encyclopedia*, Wikimedia Foundation Inc., Jan. 2, 2011, http://en.wikipedia.org/wiki/Joseph_Biederman.

10. Carey Goldberg, "Papers Reveal Push on Drug Firm Funds," *Boston Globe*, Nov. 25, 2008, http://www.boston.com/news/local/massachusetts/articles/2008/11/25/papers_reveal_push_on_drug_firm_funds/.

11. Jed Lipinski, "'Anatomy of an Epidemic': The Hidden Damage of Psychiatric Drugs," Salon, April 27, 2010, http://www.salon.com/books/feature/2010/04/27/interview_whitaker_anatomy_of_an_epidemic.

12. Whitaker, *Anatomy of an Epidemic*, 234.

13. Terry Messman, "Psychiatric Drugs: Chemical Warfare on Humans—Interview with Robert Whitaker," Natural News, Aug. 27, 2005, http://www.naturalnews.com/011353.html#ixzz1DSN8c6zN.

14. Stephanie Saul, "Merck Wrote Drug Studies for Doctors," *New York Times*, April 16, 2008, http://www.nytimes.com/2008/04/16/business/16vioxx.html.

15. John Dorschner, "UM Professor Accused of Submitting Ghostwritten Textbook," *Miami Herald*, Dec. 3, 2010, http://www.miamiherald.com/2010/12/03/1954823/um-professor-accused-of-submitting.html.

16. Dorschner, "UM Professor Accused."

17. Marc A. Rodwin, "Drug Advertising, Continuing Medical Education, and Physician Prescribing Review: A Historical Review and Reform Proposal," *Conundrums and Controversies in Mental Illness* (Winter 2010), http://www.law.suffolk.edu/faculty/addinfo/rodwin/DrugAdsCME+MDprescribingReformProposal.pdf.

18. Ibid., 809.

19. Ibid., 811.

20. Vera Hassner Sharav, "BMJ & Lancet Wedded to Merck CME Partnership," Alliance for Human Research Protection, Feb. 14, 2011, http://www.ahrp.org/cms/content/view/766/55/.

21. Adriane Fugh-Berman and Shahram Ahari, "Following the Script: How Drug Reps Make Friends and Influence Doctors," *PLoS Medicine* 4 (2007), http://www.plosmedicine.org/article/info:doi/10.1371/journal.pmed.0040150.

22. "New Jersey Youth Get Rapid Access to Mental Health Services," Bristol-Myers Squibb, Dec. 12, 2008, http://investor.bms.com/phoenix.zhtml?c=106664&p=irol-newsArticle_Print&ID=1235521&highlight=.

23. Whitaker, *Anatomy of an Epidemic*, 317.

24. Ibid.

25. "National Alliance on Mental Illness," *Wikipedia the Free Encyclopedia*, Wikimedia Foundation Inc., 2008, http://en.wikipedia.org/wiki/National_Alliance_for_the_Mentally_Ill.

26. Gardiner Harris, "Drug Makers Are Advocacy Group's Biggest Donors," *New York Times*, Oct. 21, 2009, http://www.nytimes.com/2009/10/22/health/22nami.html.

27. Dr. Joseph Mercola, "Drug Companies Triple Money on Direct-to-Consumer Drug Ads," Mercola, Feb. 27, 2002, http://articles.mercola.com/sites/articles/archive/2002/02/27/drug-ads-part-two.aspx.

28. Robert Whitaker, "Summing Up the NIMH Trials: Evidence of an Effective Paradigm of Care?" *Mad in America*, May 28, 2010, http://www.psychologytoday.com/blog/mad-in-america/201005/summing-the-nimh-trials-evidence-effective-paradigm-care.

29. M. Asif Ishmail, "Drug Lobby Second to None: How the Pharmaceutical Industry Gets Its Way in Washington," The Center for Public Integrity, July 7, 2005, http://projects.publicintegrity.org/rx/report.aspx?aid=723.

30. Bara Vaida and Christopher Weaver, "Drug Lobby's Tax Filings Reveal Health Debate," Kaiser Health News, Dec. 1, 2010, http://www.kaiserhealthnews.org/Stories/2010/December/01/phrma-drug-lobbying-health-reform.aspx.

31. Kathleen Blanchard, "Pharma Spends 40 Million on Lobbying," EmaxHealth, July 24, 2004, http://www.emaxhealth.com/1020/10/32434/pharma-spends-40-million-lobbying.html.

32. Emad Mekay, "What 800 Million Buys on Capitol Hill," Common Dreams, July 8, 2005, http://www.commondreams.org/headlines05/0708-03.htm.

33. Ed Silverman, "Bart Stupack: From Pharma Watchdog to Lobbyist," Pharmalot, Apr. 11, 2011, http://www.pharmalot.com/2011/04/bart-stupak-from-pharma-watchdog-to-lobbyist/.

34. Gregory M. Lamb, "A New Corporate Villain—Drugmakers?" *Christian Science Monitor*, Sept. 20, 2004, http://www.csmonitor.com/2004/0920/p11s02-ussc.html.

35. Vera Hassner Sharav, "Children Rx ADHD Drugs 7.4 Times Increased Risk of Sudden Death," Alliance for Human Research Protection, Jun. 17, 2009, http://www.ahrp.org/cms/content/view/609/52/.

36. Thomas Sullivan, "Prescription Drug Sakes 2009—IMS Data," Policy and Medicine, Apr. 7, 2010, http://www.policymed.com/2010/04/prescription-drug-sales-2009—ims-data.html.

37. Ed Silverman, "Evidence for Abilify & Bipolar Disorder Is Debated," Pharmalot, May 4, 2011, http://www.pharmalot.com/2011/05/evidence-for-abilify-bipolar-disorder-is-debated/.

38. Jim Edwards, "1,000 a Pop: How Forest Labs Bribed Doctors to Prescribe Antidepressants to Kids," BNET, Sept. 15, 2010, http://www.bnet.com/blog/drug-business/1000-a-pop-how-forest-labs-bribed-doctors-to-prescribe-antidepressants-to-kids/5753.

39. Ibid.

40. Duff Wilson, "Side Effects May Include Lawsuits," *New York Times*, Oct. 2, 2010, http://www.nytimes.com/2010/10/03/business/03psych.html.

41. Ibid.

42. Ibid.

43. Breeding and Philo, "Relentless and Tragic Marketing."

44. Patricia Wen, "Some in Congress Look at Incentives in Disability Benefit," *Boston Globe,* Jan. 18, 2011, http://www.boston.com/news/local/massachusetts/articles/2011/01/18/some_in_congress_look_at_incentives_in_disability_benefit/?s_campaign=8315.

45. Breeding and Philo, "Relentless and Tragic Marketing."

46. John Kelly "Psyche Meds in Jails," Youth Today, Oct. 1, 2010, http://youthtoday.org/view_article.cfm?article_id=4344.

47. Evelyn Pringle, "Suicide Prevention Drug Pushing Racket—Part II," Natural News, Aug. 21, 2009, http://www.naturalnews.com/026895_suicide_drugs_suicides.html.

48. Vince Boehm, "The Dark Underbelly of Antipsychotics," Beyond Meds, May 22, 2010, http://bipolarblast.wordpress.com/2010/05/22/the-dark-underbelly-of%c2%a0antipsychotics/.

49. "Are Foster Kids Overmedicated?" *Need to Know,* PBS, Texas, Jan. 7, 2011.

CHAPTER 5

1. Cooper, W. O., Arbogast, P. G., Ding, H., Hisckson, G. B., Fuchs, C., & Ray, W. A. (2006). Trends in prescribing of antipsychotic medications for U.S. children. *Ambulatory Pediatrics, 6*(2), 79–83; Crystal, S., Olfson, M., Huang, C., Pincus, H., & Gerhard, T. (2009). Broadened use of atypical antipsychotics: Safety, effectiveness, and policy challenges. *Health Affairs, 28,* 770–781; Olfson, M., Blanco, C., Liu, L., Moreno, C., & Laje, G. (2006). National trends in outpatient treatment of children and adolescents with antipsychotic drugs. *Archives of General Psychiatry, 63*(6), 679–685; Moreno, C., Laje, G., Blanco, C., Jiang, H., Schmidt, A., & Olfson, M. (2007). National trends in the outpatient diagnosis and treatment of bipolar disorder in youth. *Archives of General Psychiatry, 64,* 1032–1039; Patel, N. C., Crismon, M. L., Hoagwood, K., Johnsrud, M. T., Rascati, K. L., Wilson, J. P., & Jensen, P. S. (2005). Trends in the use of typical and atypical antipsychotics in children and adolescents. *Journal of the American Academy of Child and Adolescent Psychiatry, 44*(6), 548–556; Olfson, M., Crystal, S., Huang, C., & Gerhard, T. (2010). Trends in antipsychotic drug use by very young, privately insured children. *Journal of the American Academy of Child Psychiatry, 49,* 13–23.

2. Cooper, W. O., Arbogast, P. G., Ding, H., Hisckson, G. B., Fuchs, C., & Ray, W. A. (2006). Trends in prescribing of antipsychotic medications for U.S. children. *Ambulatory Pediatrics, 6*(2), 79–83; Pathak, P., West, D., Martin, B., Helm, & Henderson, C. (2010). Evidence-based use of second-generation antipsychotics in a state Medicaid pediatric population, 2001–2005. *Psychiatric Service, 61,* 123–129.

3. According to our reviews, there are no studies supporting polypharmacy for this population. dosReis, S., Zito, J. M., Safer, D. J., Gardner, J. F., Puccia, K. B., & Owens, P. L. (2005). Multiple psychotropic medication for youths: A two-state comparison. *Journal of Child & Adolescent Psychopharmacology, 15*(1), 68–77.

4. Olfson, Crystal, Huang, & Gerhard. Trends in antipsychotic drug use by very young, privately insured children.

5. Pathak, West, Martin, Helm, & Henderson. Evidence-based use of second-generation antipsychotics in a state Medicaid pediatric population, 2001–2005.

6. Crystal et al., Broadened use of atypical antipsychotics.

7. Kelly, J. (2010, October 1). Psych meds in jails. *Youth Today*. Retrieved from http://youthtoday.org/view_article.cfm?article_id=4344

8. Norcross, J. C., Beutler, L. E., & Levant, R. F. (2006). Prologue. In J. C. Norcross, L. E. Beutler & R. L. Levant (Eds.), *Evidence-based practices in mental health: Debate and dialogue on the Fundamental Questions* (pp. 3–12). Washington, DC: American Psychological Association; Benjamin, L. T., & Baker, D. B. (Eds.). (2000). History of psychology: The Boulder Conference. *American Psychologist, 55,* 233–254.

9. APA Working Group on Psychoactive Medications for Children and Adolescents. (2006). *Report of the Working Group on Psychoactive Medications for Children and Adolescents. Psychopharmacological, psychosocial, and combined interventions for childhood disorders: Evidence base, contextual factors, and future directions.* Washington, DC: American Psychological Association.

10. Kowatch, R. A., Fristad, M. A., Birmaher, B., Wagner, K. D., Findling, R. L., Hellander, M., & Child Psychiatric Workgroup on Bipolar Disorder. (2005). Treatment guidelines for children and adolescents with bipolar disorder. *Journal of the American Academy of Child & Adolescent Psychiatry, 44*(3), 213–235.

11. Correll, C. U., Manu, P., Olshanskiy, V., Napolitano, B., Kane, J. M., & Malhotra, K. A. (2009). Cardiometabolic risk of second-generation medications during first-time use in children and adolescents. *JAMA, 302*(16), 1765–2322.

12. Wilson, D. (2009, October 28). Rapid weight gain associated linked to antipsychotic drugs. *New York Times*, p. B.1.

13. Varley, C. K., & McClellan, J. (2009). Implications of marked weight gain associated with atypical antipsychotic medications in children and adolescents. *JAMA, 302*(16), 1811–1812.

14. Woods, S. W., Morgenstern, H., Saksa, J. R., Walsh, B. C., Sullivan, M. C., Money, R., . . . Glazer, W. M. (2010). Incidence of tardive dyskinesia with atypical versus conventional antipsychotic medications: A prospective cohort study. *The Journal of Clinical Psychiatry, 71*(4), 463–474.

15. http://www.medscape.com/viewarticle/717316?src=emailthis

16. Sparks, J., Duncan, B. L., Cohen, D., & Antonuccio, D. (2010). Psychiatric drugs and common factors: An evaluation of risks and benefits for clinical practice. In B. L. Duncan, S. D. Miller, B. E. Wampold & M. A. Hubble (Eds.), *The heart and soul of change: Delivering what works* (2nd ed., pp. 199–236). Washington, DC: American Psychological Association.

17. Sikich, L., Frazier, J. A., McClellan, J., Findling, R. L., Vitiello, B., Ritz, L., et al. (2008). Double-blind comparison of first-and second-generation antipsychotics in early-onset schizophrenia and schizoaffective disorder: Findings from the treatment of early-onset schizophrenia spectrum disorders (TEOSS) study. *American Journal of Psychiatry, 165,* 1420–1431; Findling, R., Johnson, J., McClellan, J., Frazier, J., Vitiello, B., Hamer, R., et al. (2010). Double-blind maintenance safety and effectiveness findings from the Treatment of Early-Onset Schizophrenia Spectrum (TEOSS) study. *Journal of the American Academy of Child Adolescent Psychiatry, 49,* 583–594.

18. These percentages must be understood in light of the study's definition of response (Clinical Global Impression, CGI, score of at least 2, much improved, plus a > 20% reduction in baseline on the Positive and Negative Syndrome Scale, PANSS). According to an analysis of cutoff and response scores for the PANSS (see

Findling et al. in note 17), reduction of PANSS of > 28% correlates with CGI "minimally improved." The low cutoff on the PANSS in this trial calls into question the clinical meaningfulness of the response rates reported.

19. Findling, et al. Double-blind maintenance safety and effectiveness findings from the Treatment of Early-Onset Schizophrenia Spectrum (TEOSS) study, p. 584.

20. Critical readers who want to evaluate the psychiatric drug trial literature can review Sparks et al. (2010) for a detailed description of a five-flaws analysis.

21. Findling, R., Robb, A., Nyila, M., Forbes, R. A., Jin, N., Ivanova, S., et al. (2008). A multiple-center, randomized, double-blind, placebo-controlled study of oral aripiprazole for treatment of adolescents with schizophrenia. *American Journal of Psychiatry, 165*(11), 1432–1441.

22. Study authors reported a difference between placebo and drug groups in the overall PQLES-Q score. The overall score is a separate, one-item score. As such, it is not valid or reliable as an indicator of patient status or change.

23. Wilson, D. (2010, September 2). Child's ordeal reveals risks of psychiatric drugs in young. *New York Times*, p. A.1.

24. APA Working Group on Psychoactive Medications for Children and Adolescents, p. 126.

25. Lyotard, J. (1979). *The postmodern condition: A report on knowledge.* Minneapolis: University of Minnesota Press.

26. Duncan, B., Miller, S., & Sparks, J. (2004). *The heroic client: A revolutionary way to improve effectiveness through client-directed, outcome-informed therapy.* San Francisco: Jossey-Bass; Sparks, J. A., Duncan, B. L. & Murphy, J. J. (2007). Medication, children, & schools. In J. J. Murphy & B. L. Duncan (authors), *Brief outcome informed intervention in the schools.* New York: The Guilford Press.

27. IMS Health. (2010). IMS Health reports U.S. sales grew 5.1 percent in 2009, to 300.3 billion. Retrieved from http://www.imshealth.com/portal/site/ims health/menuitem.a46c6d4df3db4b3d88f611019418c22a/?vgnextoid=d690a27e9d 5b7210VgnVCM100000ed152ca2RCRD

28. Weber, T., & Ornstein, C. (2010, November 1). Dollars for docs: Who's on pharma's top-paid list? Retrieved from http://www.propublica.org/article/ profiles-of-the-top-earners-in-dollar-for-docs

29. Wazana, A. (2000). Physicians and the pharmaceutical industry: Is a gift ever just a gift? *JAMA, 283*(3), 373–380.

30. Angell, M. (2000). Is academic medicine for sale? *New England Journal of Medicine, 341*(20), 1516–1518.

31. Horton, R. (2004). The dawn of McScience. *New York Review of Books 51*(4): 7–9.

32. Wilson, D. (2010, November 29). Drug maker wrote book under 2 doctors' names, documents say. *New York Times*, p. B.3.

33. Heres, S., Davis, J., Maino, K., Jetzinger, E., Kissling, W., & Leucht, S. (2006). Why olanzapine beats risperidone, risperidone beats quetiapine, and comparison studies of second-generation antipsychotics. *American Journal of Psychiatry, 163*(2), 185–194.

34. Vedantam, S. (2006, April 12). Comparison of schizophrenia drugs often favors firm funding study. *The Washington Post*, p. A01.

35. Bekelman, J. E., Li, Y., & Gross, C. P. (2003). Scope and impact of financial conflicts of interest in biomedical research: A systematic review. *JAMA, 289*(4), 454–465.

36. Melander, H., Ahlqvist-Rastad, J., Meijer, G., & Beermann, B. (2003). Evidence b(i)ased medicine—selective reporting from studies sponsored by pharmaceutical

industry: review of studies in new drug applications. *British Medical Journal, 326*(7400), 1171–1173; Turner, E. H., Matthews, A. M., Linardatos, E., Tell, R. A., & Rosenthal, R. (2008). Selective publication of antidepressant trials and its influence on apparent efficacy. *New England Journal of Medicine, 358,* 252–260; Wieseler, B., McGaura, N., & Kaiser, T. (2010). Finding studies on reboxetine: A tale of hide and seek. *British Medical Journal, 341,* c4942.

37. Angell, M. (2009). Drug companies and doctors: A story of corruption. *New York Review of Books.* Retrieved from http://www.nybooks.com/articles/archives/2009/jan/15/drug-companies-doctorsa-story-of-corruption/?page=1

38. Whitaker, R. (2010). *Anatomy of and epidemic: Magic bullet, psychiatric drugs, and the astonishing rise of mental illness in America.* New York: Crown Publishers, p. 326.

39. Harris, G. (2008, November 19). Use of antipsychotics in children is criticized. *New York Times,* p. A.20.

40. Harris, G. (2008, November 25). Ties between child psychiatry center drug maker. *New York Times,* p. A.22.

41. Kowalczyk, L. (2009, March 21). Senator broadens inquiry into psychiatrist. *Boston Globe,* p. B.1, Metro.

42. http://www.medscape.com/viewarticle/727430

43. Findling, Robb, Nyila, Forbes, Jin, Ivanova, et al. A multiple-center, randomized, double-blind, placebo-controlled study of oral aripiprazole for treatment of adolescents with schizophrenia.

44. Of note, not only were Findling and the second author, Robb, listed as receiving research support from, acting as consultant to, and/or serving on a speakers bureau for Bristol-Myers Squibb/Otsuka, the manufacturer of Abilify, but the remaining nine authors were listed as employees of that company, p. 1432.

45. Willman, D. (2003, December 7). Stealth merger: Drug companies and government medical research. *Los Angeles Times,* p. A.1; Willman, D. (2005, July 14). NIH inquiry shows widespread ethical lapses, lawmaker says. *Los Angeles Times,* p. A.23.

46. Whitaker. *Anatomy of and epidemic.*

47. Lurie, P., Almeida, C. M., Stine, N., Stine, A., & Wolfe, (2006). Financial conflict of interest disclosure and voting patterns at Food and Drug Administration Drug Advisory Committee meetings. *Journal of the American Medical Association, 295*(16), 26, 1921–1928.

48. Cosgrove, L., Krimsky, S., Vijayaraghavan, M., & Schneider, L. (2006). Financial ties between DSM-IV panel members and the pharmaceutical industry. *Psychotherapy Psychosomatics, 75,* 154–160.

49. Choudhry, N. K., Stelfox, H. T., & Detsky, A. S. (2002). Relationships between authors of clinical practice guidelines and the pharmaceutical industry. *JAMA, 287*(5), 612–617.

50. Hughes, C. W., Emslie, G. J., Crismon, M. L., Posner, K., Birmaher, B., Ryan, N., et al. (2007). Texas Children's Medication Algorithm Project: Update from Texas Consensus Conference Panel on Medication Treatment for childhood major depressive disorder. *Journal of the American Academy of Child & Adolescent Psychiatry, 46*(6), 667–686.

51. Antonuccio, D. O., Danton, W. G., & McClanahan, T. M. (2003). Psychology in the prescription era: Building a firewall between marketing and science. *American Psychologist, 58*(12), 1028–1043.

52. McClellan, J., Kowatch, R., Findling, R. L. & Workgroup on Quality Issues. (2007). Practice parameters for the assessment and treatment of children and

adolescents with bipolar disorder. *Journal of the American Academy of Child & Adolescent Psychiatry, 46*(1), 107–125.

53. AAMFT consumer update: Mental illness in children. Retrieved from http://www.aamft.org/families/Consumer_Updates/MentalIllnessinChildren.asp

54. AAMFT consumer update: Bipolar disorder in children and adolescents. Retrieved from http://www.aamft.org/families/Consumer_Updates/BipolarDisorderinChildrenandAdolescents.asp

55. We acknowledge that there are psychiatrists who decry the wholesale takeover of their field by the pharmaceutical industry. Our term *psychiatric establishment* refers to the body of pro-drug training, literature, and research produced and promulgated by the field of psychiatry in America and its alliance with drug companies through these activities as discussed throughout this chapter.

56. Our recommended guidelines in no way preclude any action necessary on the part of a clinician to prevent client self-harm, harm to others, or duty to warn. However, we challenge clinicians not to assume automatically that antipsychotic medications are a preferred choice in these circumstances.

57. For a primer of how to read clinical trial research using a five-flaws analysis, visit

58. Sparks, Duncan, Cohen, & Antonuccio. Psychiatric drugs and common factors.

59. Providing information regarding a risk-benefit profile of antipsychotics to the parents and caretakers of children and adolescents does not preclude identifying other sources of information that may be helpful, as recommended in step 6.

60. A detailed description of how to systematically collect and utilize child, youth, and family feedback throughout treatment to improve outcomes can be found at

61. Nonmedical practitioners can also advocate for ethical practice guidelines for prescribers, as recommended by Duncan and Antonuccio (2010): (1) full disclosure of risks, (2) psychosocial options tried first, (3) no nonempirically supported practices, (4) privileging patient-rated measures in practice and research, (5) no pharmaceutical perks, and (6) the creation of an unbiased database to inform practitioners and clients. (Duncan, B., & Antonuccio, D. (2010). *A patient bill of rights for psychotropic prescription: A call for a higher standard of care.* Manuscript submitted for publication.)

62. Duncan, B. L. (2010). *On becoming a better therapist.* Washington, DC: American Psychological Association.

CHAPTER 6

1. Gottstein, J. (2010). Ethical and moral obligations arising from revelations of pharmaceutical company dissembling." *Ethical Human Psychology and Psychiatry 12*(1), 22–29.

2. Nowak, M. (2008). *Interim report of the Special Rapporteur on torture and other cruel, inhuman or degrading treatment or punishment.* United Nations General Assembly, 16. ("The Special Rapporteur notes that forced and non-consensual administration of psychiatric drugs, and in particular of neuroleptics, for the treatment of a mental condition needs to be closely scrutinized. Depending on the circumstances

of the case, the suffering inflicted and the effects upon the individual's health may constitute a form of torture or ill-treatment.")

3. American Psychological Association. (2006). *Resolution against torture and other cruel, inhuman, and degrading treatment or punishment;* American Psychological Association. (2007). *Reaffirmation of the American Psychological Association position against torture and other cruel, inhuman, or degrading treatment or punishment and its application to individuals defined in the United States Code as "enemy combatants."*

4. See, e.g., *Columbia Physical Therapy v. Benton Franklin Orthopedic Associates,* 228 P.3d 1260, 1266 (Washington 2010), quoting Revised Code of Washington § 18.71.030(4).

5. 47 N.C. App. 680.687 (NC App. 1980), *overruled on other grounds.* See, also, Indiana Code § 25–22–5–1–2(a)(18); *Columbia Physical Therapy, Inc., P.S., v. Benton Franklin Orthopedic Associates,* 228 P.3d 1260, 1266 (Washington 2010).

6. National Association of Social Workers. (2008). *Code of ethics of the National Association of Social Workers, National Association of Social Workers, 1996, revised 2008.*

7. http://criticalthinkrx.org

8. *DeShaney v. Winnebago County Dep't of Soc. Servs.,* 489 U.S. 189, 199–200 (1989).

9. See, *Whalen v. Allers,* 302 F.Supp.2d 194, 203–204 (S.D.N.Y. 2003) for a discussion of children's rights to enforce their own constitutional rights.

10. See, *American Academy of Pediatrics v. Lungren,* 940 P.2d 797, 814–16, 819 (1997); *In re T.W.,* 551 So.2d 1186, 1194 (Fla.1989); *Planned Parenthood of Central N.J. v. Farmer,* 165 N.J. 609, 762 A.2d 620, 626, 631–39 (2000); *State v. Planned Parenthood of Alaska,* 35 P.3d 30, 41 (Alaska 2001).

11. Camp, A. (2011). A mistreated epidemic: State and federal failure to adequately regulate psychotropic medications prescribed to children in foster care. 83 *Temple L. Rev.* 101.

12. Dawsey, D. (2011, March 28). Was a Detroit mother right to resist efforts by Child Protective Services, police to take her child? *MLive.com.*

13. *In re G.K.,* 993 A.2d 558 (D.C. Cir. 2010).

14. Burton, A. (2010). "They use it like candy": How the prescription of psychotropic drugs to state-involved children violates international law. 35 *Brooklyn Journal of International Law* 453.

15. *Id.,* at 470.

16. *Id.*

17. Doek, J. E. (2006). What does the Children's Convention require? 20 *Emory International Law Rev.* 199.

18. Stahl, R. M. (2007). "Don't forget about me": Implementing Article 12 of the United Nations Convention on the Rights of the Child. 24 *Ariz. J. Int'l & Comp. L.* 803.

19. *Law Project for Psychiatric Rights, Inc. v. State of Alaska et al.,* Case No. 3AN 08–10115CI, Superior Court, Third Judicial District, State of Alaska.

20. The Amended Complaint is available at http://psychrights.org/States/Alaska/PsychRightsvAlaska/PsychRightsvAlaskaKidDruggingComplaintAmended.pdf

21. Alaska Statutes 47.12.084(e), 47.12.150(a), & 47.14.100(d)(1).

22. 42 United States Code §1983.

23. Crystal, S., Olfson, M., Huang, C., Pincus, H., & Gerhard, T. (2009). Broadened use of atypical antipsychotics: Safety, effectiveness, and policy challenges. *Health Affairs,* 28, 770–781; "Are foster kids overmedicated?" *Need to Know,* PBS, Texas, Jan. 7, 2011.

24. 42 United States Code § 1396r-8(k)(3); § 1396r-8(k)(6); & 42 USC § 1396r-8(g)(1)(B)(i).

25. The Medically Accepted Indications Chart is available at http://psych rights.org/Education/ModelQuiTam/PediatricPsychotropicMedicallyAccept edIndications.pdf

26. 31 United States Code §3729 et. seq.

27. 31 USC §3729(a)(1).

28. 31 U.S.C. §3729(b)(1)(a)

29. Heckler v. Community Health Services, 467 U.S. 51, 63–64 (1984).

30. United States v. Nazon, 940 F.2d 255, 259 (7th Cir. 1991); U.S. v. Cooperative Grain & Supply, 476 F.2d 47, 55–60 (8th Cir. 1973)

31. Kesselheim, A., et al. (2011). Strategies and practices in off-label marketing of pharmaceuticals: A retrospective analysis of whistleblower complaints. PLOS Medicine,

32. The Model Complaint is available at http://psychrights.org/Education/ModelQuiTam/PsychRightsModelQuiTamComplaint.pdf

33. U.S. ex rel Law Project for Psychiatric Rights v. Matsutani, et al., Case No. 3:09-cv-0080 & U.S. ex rel Griffin v. Martino, et al., 3:09-cv-246, United States District Court for the District of Alaska.

34. . U.S. ex rel. Nicholson v. Spigelman, et al., Case No 10-cv-3361, United States District Court for the Northern District of Illinois.

35. 31 United States Code § 3730(b).

36. Page 21 in Docket No. 163, United States ex rel Law Project for Psychiatric Rights v. Matsutani et al., No. 3:09-cv-80, and Docket No. 26 in U.S. ex rel Griffin v. Martino, Family Centered Services and Safeway, No. 3:09-cv-246, available at http://psychrights.org/States/Alaska/Matsutani/163–100924Order2DismissMatsutani.pdf

37. Griffin and Law Project for Psychiatric Rights v. Matsutani et al., Case No. 10–35887, United States Court of Appeals for the Ninth Circuit.

38. 42 United States Code §10801, et seq.

CHAPTER 7

1. Whitaker, R. (2010). Anatomy of an epidemic. New York: Crown.

2. Lieberman, A. F., & Van Horn, P. (2008). Psychotherapy with infants and young children. New York: Guilford Press.

3. Bowlby, J. (1969, 1975, 1980). Attachment and loss (3 vols.). New York: Basic Books.

4. Fraiberg, S. (1980). Clinical studies in infant mental health. New York: Basic Books.

5. Lieberman and Van Horn, Psychotherapy.

6. Schore, A. N. (1994). Affect regulation and the origin of the self. New Jersey: Lawrence Erlbaum.

7. Siegel, D. J. (1999). The developing mind. New York: Guilford Press; Siegel, D. J. (2004). Parenting from the inside out. New York: Jeremy P. Tarcher/Penguin; Siegel, D. J., Fosha, D., & Solomon, M. F. (2009). The healing power of emotion. New York: W.W. Norton; Perry, B. D., & Szalavitz, M. (2006). The boy who was raised as a dog. New York: Basic Books; Perry, B. D., & Szalavitz, M. (2010). Born for love. New

York: HarperCollins; Stern, D. N. (1985). *The interpersonal world of the infant.* New York: Basic Books.

8. Coles, R. (1989). *The call of stories.* Boston: Houghton Mifflin Company.

9. The title "The Unfinished Copernican Revolution" is taken from a paper by that name written by the French psychoanalyst Jean Laplance (1999).

10. Lewis, M., Brown, T. E., Hooven, M., & O'Hare, E. (1978, Spring). Medication in residential treatment. *Child Psychiatry and Human Development, 8*(3).

11. Olfman, S. (Ed.). (2007). *Bipolar children.* Westport, CT: Praeger Publishers.

12. Sprinson, J. S. & Berrick, K. (2009). *Relationship-based, behavioral intervention with vulnerable children and families.* New York: Oxford University.

CHAPTER 8

1. Duncan, et al., *The Heart & Soul of Change.*

2. Moynihan and Cassells, *Selling Sickness.*

3. Ibid.

4. Publication of the *DSM-IV* brings in about $60 million dollars in revenue for the APA.

5. Whitehead, "An Interview with Allen Jones." The creators of the drug use protocol known as TEXAS MEDICATION ALGORITHM PROGRAM (TMAP) claim they used "scientific evidence" to establish the safety and effectiveness of the psychiatric drugs on their list "best practice drugs." However, TMAP personnel tampered with the research results through a process known as "Retrospective Analysis." Patients previously treated with the new antipsychotic medications being pushed were researched, and files showing positive results were selected out and reported on. TMAP research "confirmed" that the new drugs were safer and more effective than the older treatments. TMAP employees referred to their algorithm as an "Evidence-Based Best Practice." However, the guidelines promoted by the program were based on "opinions, not data," and "most of the guidelines' authors have received financial support from the pharmaceutical industry." TMAP drugs were selected by an "expert consensus process" rigged to promoted special interests. "A project management team tied to the drug industry selected other doctors whose opinions were then analyzed or accessed by TMAP." That rigged consensus determined these drugs were safer and more effective. Of the 55 doctors pooled for the first schizophrenia consensus, 27 had financial ties to the pharmaceutical industry. The drugs on the TMAP list were all new drugs still "on patent" and cost 100 times more than older drugs whose patents had expired. Later, a CHILDRENS' MEDICATION ALGORITHM PROGRAM (CMAP) was developed in Texas in the same way.

6. Pelham (2009) in Midkiff and Wyatt, "Has Behavioral Science Tumbled through the Looking Glass?"

7. Wikipedia, http://en.wikipedia.org/wiki/Arnold_van_Gennep.

8. Van Gennep, *The Rites of Passage.*

9. Wiener, N. (1948) *Cybernetics: Or Control and Communication in the Animal and the Machine.* Cambridge. MA, MIT Press.

10. V. Turner, (1969) *The Ritual Process: Structure and Anti-Structure.* 1995 paperback Aldine Transaction.

11. V. Turner, 1995.

12. E. Turner, personal communication, 1996.

13. J. Haley, personal communication, 1977.

CHAPTER 9

1. Blader, J. C. (2010, October). *Larger growth in U.S. acute-care hospitalization for psychiatric disorders among youth than adults, 1996–2007.* Poster presented at the Annual Meeting of the American Academy of Child and Adolescent Psychiatry, NY.

2. Paston, P. N., & Reuben, C. A. (2008). Diagnosed attention deficit hyperactivity disorder and learning disability: United States, 2004–2006. National Center for Health Statistics. *Vital and Health Statistics, 10*(237); Centers for Disease Control and Prevention. (2010). Increasing prevalence of parent-reported attention-deficit/hyperactivity disorder among children—United States, 2003 and 2007. *Morbidity and Mortality Weekly Report, 59*, 1439–1443.

3. Centers for Disease Control and Prevention. (2009). Prevalence of autism spectrum disorders—Autism and Developmental Disabilities Monitoring Network, United States, 2006. Surveillance Summaries (2006). *MMWR, 58*(No. SS-10).

4. Moreno, C., Laje, G., Blanco, C., Jiang, H., Schmidt, A. B., & Olfson, M. (2007). National trends in the outpatient diagnosis and treatment of bipolar disorder in youth. *Archives of General Psychiatry, 64*, 1032–1039.

5. For example, Olfson, M., Crystal, S., Huang, C., & Gerhard, T. (2010). Trends in antipsychotic drug use by very young, privately insured children. *Journal of the American Academy of Child and Adolescent Psychiatry, 49*, 13–23; Olfson, M., Marcus, S. C., Weissman, M. M., & Jensen, P. S. (2002). National trends in the use of psychotropic medications by children. *Journal of the American Academy of Child and Adolescent Psychiatry, 41*, 514–521.

6. Moreno et al., National trends.

7. Public Agenda. (2002). A lot easier said than done: Parents talk about raising children in today's America. Retrieved from www.publicagenda.org/spe cials/parents/parents.htm

8. Vandivere, S., Gallagher, M., & Moore, K. A. (2004). *Changes in children's well-being and family environments. Snapshots of America's families III, No. 10.* New York: Urban Institute. Retrieved from www.urban.org/url.cfm?ID=310912

9. Jensen, P. S., & Hoagwood, K. (1997). The book of names: DSM-IV in context. *Development and Psychopathology, 9*, 231–249; Jensen, Hoagwood, & Zitner, 2006. What's in a name? Problems vs. prospects in current diagnostic approaches. In D. Cicchetti & D. J. Cohen (Eds.), *Developmental psychopathology: Theory and method.*

10. See, for example, Goodyer, I. M. (2006). The hypothalamic-pituitary-adrenal axis: Cortisol, DHEA, and psychopathology. In M. E. Garralda & M. Flament (Eds.), *Working with children and adolescents: An evidence-based approach to risk and resilience.* Lanham, MD: Jason Aronson; Hebebrand, J., Reichwald, K., Schimmelmann, B.G., & Hinney, A. (2006). Identifying genes underlying child and adolescent psychiatric disorders. In M. E. Garralda & M. Flament (Eds.), *Working with children and adolescents: An evidence-based approach to risk and resilience.* Lanham, MD: Jason Aronson; Kim, Y. (Ed). (2009). *Handbook of behavior genetics.* New York: Springer.

11. Findling, R. L. (Ed.). (2008). *Clinical manual of child and adolescent psychophar-macology.* Washington, DC: American Psychiatric Publishing.

12. Rutter, M., & Sroufe, L. A. (2000). Developmental psychopathology: Concepts and challenges. *Development and Psychopathology, 12,* 265–295.

13. Cichetti, D., & Rogosch, F. A. (1996). Equifinality and multifinality in developmental psychopathology. *Development and Psychopathology, 8,* 597–600.

14. Frick, P. J., & Viding, E. (2009). Antisocial behavior from a developmental psychopathology perspective. *Development and Psychopathology, 21,* 1111–1131. See also: Cornell, A. H., & Frick, P. J. (2007). The moderating effects of parenting styles in the association between behavioral inhibition and parent-reported guilt and empathy in preschool children. *Journal of Clinical Child & Adolescent Psychology, 36,* 305–318.

15. Cicchetti, D. (2010). A developmental psychopathology perspective on bipolar disorder. In D. J. Milkiwitz (Ed.). *Understanding bipolar disorder: A developmental psychopathology perspective.* New York: Guilford.

16. Baker, J. K., Messinger, D. S., Lyons, K. K., & Grantz, C. J. (2010). A pilot study of maternal sensitivity in the context of emergent autism. *Journal of Autism and Developmental Disorders, 40,* 988–999.

17. Baker, J. K., Smith, L. E., Greenberg, J. S., Seltzer, M. M., & Taylor, J. L. (2011). Change in maternal criticism and behavior problems in adolescents and adults with autism across a 7-year period. *Journal of Family Psychology, 24,* 775–777; Smith, L. E., Greenberg, J. S., Seltzer, M. M., & Hong, J. (2008). Symptoms and behavior problems of adolescents and adults with autism: Effects of mother-child relationship quality, warmth, and praise. *American Journal on Mental Retardation, 113,* 387–402.

18. Miklowitz, D. J. (2004). The role of family systems in severe and recurrent psychiatric disorders: A developmental psychopathology view. *Development and Psychopathology, 16,* 667–688.

19. Miklowitz, D. J., Axelson, D. A., Birmaher, B., George, E. L., Taylor, D. O., Schneck, C. D., . . . Brent, D. A. (2008). Family-focused treatment for adolescents with bipolar disorder: Results of a 2-year randomized trial. *Archives of General Psychiatry, 65,* 1053–1061.

20. Bouchard, T. J. (2004). Genetic influence on human psychological traits: A survey. *Current Directions in Psychological Science, 13,* 148–151; Bouchard, T. J., & Loehlin, J. C. (2001). Genes, evolution, and personality. *Behavior Genetics, 31,* 243–274; Roisman, R., & Fraley, C. (2006). The limits of genetic influence: A behavior-genetic analysis of infant–caregiver relationship quality and temperament. *Child Development, 77,* 1656–1667; Saudino, K. J., & Cherny, S. S. (2001). Sources of continuity and change in observed temperament. In R. N. Emde & J. K. Hewitt (Eds.), *Infancy to early childhood: Genetic and environmental influences on developmental change* (pp. 89–110). New York: Oxford University Press.

21. Gregory, A. M., Eley, T. C., & Plomin, R. (2004). Exploring the association between anxiety and conduct problems in a large sample of twins age 2–4. *Journal of Abnormal Child Psychology, 32,* 111–122; Lemery, K. S., & Doelger, L. (2005). Genetic vulnerabilities to psychopathology. In B. L. Hankin & J.R.Z. Abela (Eds.), *Development of psychopathology: A vulnerability-stress perspective* (pp. 161–198). Thousand Oaks, CA: Sage.

22. Rutter, M. (2011). Biological and experiential influences on psychological development. In D. P. Keating (Ed.), *Nature and nurture in early child development* (pp. 7–44). New York: Cambridge University Press.

23. See, for example, Afifi, T. O., Brownridge, D. A., Cox, B. J., & Sareen, J. (2006). Physical punishment, childhood abuse and psychiatric disorders. *Child Abuse and Neglect, 30,* 1093–1103; Bender, H. L., Allen, J. P., McElhaney, K. B., Antonishak, J., Moore, C. M., Kelly, H. L., & Davis, S. M. (2007). Use of harsh physical discipline and developmental outcomes in adolescence. *Development and Psychopathology, 19,* 227–242; Kochanska, G., & Aksan, N. (2006). Children's conscience and self-regulation. *Journal of Personality, 74,* 1587–1617; Lynch, S. K., Turkheimer, E., D'Onofrio, B. M., Mendle, J., Emery, R. E., Slutske, W. S., & Martin, N. G. (2006). A genetically informed study of the association between harsh punishment and off-spring behavioral problems. *Journal of Family Psychology, 20,* 190–198.

24. Bridgett, D. J., Gartstein, M. A., Putnam, S. P., McKay, T., Iddins, R., Robertson, C., et al. (2009). Maternal and contextual influences and the effect of temperament development during infancy on parenting in toddlerhood. *Infant Behavior and Development, 32,* 103–116; Paulussen-Hoogeboom, M. C., Stams, G J.J.M., Hermanns, J.M.A., & Peetsma, T.T.D. (2007). Child negative emotionality and parenting from infancy to preschool: A meta-analytic review. *Developmental Psychology, 43,* 438–453; Pesonen, A.-K., Räikkönen, K., Heinonen, K., & Komsi, N. (2008). A transactional model of temperamental development: Evidence of a relationship between child temperament and maternal stress over five years. *Social Development, 17,* 326–340; van Aken, C., Junger, M., Verhoeven, M., van Aken, M.A.G., & Deković, M. (2007). The interactive effects of temperament and maternal parenting on toddlers' externalizing behaviours. *Infant and Child Development, 16,* 553–572; van den Boom, D.C., & Hoeksma, J. B. (1994). The effect of infant irritability on mother–infant interaction: A growth-curve analysis. *Developmental Psychology, 30,* 581–590.

25. Feldman, R., Greenbaum, C. W., &Yirmiya, N. (1999). Mother–infant affect synchrony as an antecedent of the emergence of self-control. *Developmental Psychology, 35,* 223–231; Raikes, H. A., Robinson, J. L., Bradley, R. H., Raikes, H. H., & Ayoub, C. C. (2007). Developmental trends in self-regulation among low-income toddlers. *Social Development, 16,* 128–149.

26. Cipriano, E. A., & Stifter, C. A. (2010). Predicting preschool effortful control from toddler temperament and parenting behavior. *Journal of Applied Developmental Psychology, 31,* 221–230; Jaffari-Bimmel, N., Juffer, F., van IJzendoorn, M. H., Bakermans-Kranenburg, M. J., & Mooijaart, A. (2006). Social development from infancy to adolescence: Longitudinal and concurrent factors in an adoption sample. *Developmental Psychology, 42,* 1143–1153.

27. Tienari, P., Wynne, L. C., Laksy, K., Moring, J., Nieminen, P., Sorri, A., et al. (2003). Genetic boundaries of the schizophrenia spectrum: Evidence from the Finnish adoptive family study of schizophrenia. *The American Journal of Psychiatry, 160,* 1587–1594; Tienari, P., Wahlberg, K. E., & Wynne, L. C. (2006). Finnish adoption study of schizophrenia: Implications for family interventions. *Families, Systems, and Health, 24,* 442–451.

28. Plomin, R. (2005). *Finding genes in child psychology and psychiatry: When are we going to be there?* Unpublished manuscript. London: King's College; Plomin, R., & Davis, O.S.P. (2009). The future of genetics in psychology and psychiatry: Microarrays, genome-wide association, and non-coding RNA. *Journal of Child Psychology and Psychiatry, 50,* 63–71.

29. Ivorra, J. L., Sanjuan, J., Jover, M., Carot, J. M., de Frutos, R., & Molto, M. D. (2010). Gene-environment interaction of child temperament. *Journal of Developmental and Behavioral Pediatrics, 31*, 545–554.

30. Bakermans-Kranenburg, M. J., & van IJzendoorn, M. H. (2007). Gene–environment interaction of the dopamine D4 receptor (DRD4) and observed maternal insensitivity predicting externalizing behavior in preschoolers. *Developmental Psychobiology, 48*, 406–409.

31. Bakermans-Kranenburg, M. J., & van IJzendoorn, M. H. (2011). Differential susceptibility to rearing environment depending on dopamine-related genes: New evidence and a meta-analysis. *Development and Psychopathology, 23*, 39–52.

32. Gray, M. R., & Steinberg, L. (1999). Unpacking authoritative parenting: Reassessing a multidimensional construct. *Journal of Marriage and the Family, 61*, 574–587; Hart, C. H., Newell, L. D., & Olsen, S. F. (2003). Parenting skills and social/communicative competence in childhood. In J. O. Greene & B. R. Burleson (Eds.), *Handbook of communication and social interaction skills* (pp. 753–797). Hillsdale, NJ: Erlbaum; Russell, A., Mize, J., & Bissaker, K. (2002). Parent–child relationships. In P. K. Smith & C. H. Hart (Eds.), *Handbook of childhood social development* (pp. 205–222). Oxford, UK: Blackwell.

33. Kochanska, G., Gross, J. N., Lin, M.-H., & Nichols, K. E. (2002). Guilt in young children: Development, determinants, and relations with broader system standards. *Child Development, 73*, 461–482; Fowles, D. C., & Kochanska, G. (2000). Temperament as a moderator of pathways to conscience in children: The contribution of electrodermal activity. *Psychophysiology, 37*, 863–872; Kochanska, G. (1997). Multiple pathways to conscience for children with different temperaments: From toddlerhood to age 5. *Developmental Psychology, 33*, 228–240.

34. Baumrind, D., & Black, A. E. (1967). Child care practices anteceding three patterns of preschool behavior. *Genetic Psychology Monographs, 75*, 43–88; Gray and Steinberg, Unpacking authoritative parenting; Herman, M. R., Dornbusch, S. M., Herron, M. C., & Herting, J. R. (1997). The influence of family regulation, connection, and psychological autonomy on six measures of adolescent functioning. *Journal of Adolescent Research, 12*, 34–67; Luster, T., & McAdoo, H. (1996). Family and child influences on educational attainment: A secondary analysis of the High/Scope Perry Preschool data. *Developmental Psychology, 32*, 26–39; Mackey, K., Arnold, M. K., & Pratt, M. W. (2001). Adolescents' stories of decision making in more and less authoritative families: Representing the voices of parents in narrative. *Journal of Adolescent Research, 16*, 243–268; Steinberg, L. D., Darling, N. E., & Fletcher, A. C. (1995). Authoritative parenting and adolescent development: An ecological journey. In P. Moen, G. H. Elder, Jr. & K. Luscher (Eds.), *Examining lives in context* (pp. 423–466). Washington, DC: American Psychological Association.

35. Steinberg, L. (2001). We know some things: Parent–adolescent relationships in retrospect and prospect. *Journal of Research on Adolescence, 11*, 1–19; Chen, X., Dong, Q., & Zhou, H. (1997). Authoritative and authoritarian parenting practices and social and school performance in Chinese children. *International Journal of Behavioral Development, 21*, 855–873; Chen, X., Liu, M., & Li, D. (2000). Parental warmth, control, and indulgence and their relations to adjustment in Chinese children: A longitudinal study. *Journal of Family Psychology, 14*, 401–419; Mantzicopouilos, P. Y., & Oh-Hwang, Y. (1998). The relationship of psychosocial maturity to parenting quality and intellectual ability for American and Korean adolescents. *Contemporary Educational Psychology, 23*, 195–206.

36. Rohner, R. P., & Rohner, E. C. (1981). Parental acceptance-rejection and parental control: Cross-cultural codes. *Ethnology, 20,* 245–260.

37. Pettit, G. S., Bates, J. E., & Dodge, K. A. (1997). Supportive parenting, ecological context, and children's adjustment: A seven-year longitudinal study. *Child Development, 68,* 908–923.

38. Straus, M. A., & Stewart, J. H. (1999). Corporal punishment by American parents: National data on prevalence, chronicity, severity, and duration, in relation to child and family characteristics. *Clinical Child and Family Psychology Review, 2,* 55–70

39. Gershoff, E. T. (2002). Corporal punishment by parents and associated child behaviors and experiences: A meta-analytic and theoretical review. *Psychological Bulletin, 128,* 539–579.

40. Brezina, T. (1999). Teenage violence toward parents as an adaptation to family strain: Evidence from a national survey of male adolescents. *Youth & Society, 30,* 416–444; Gershoff, E. T. (2002). Corporal punishment by parents and associated child behaviors and experiences: A meta-analytic and theoretical review. *Psychological Bulletin, 128,* 539–579.

41. Lansford, J. E., Criss, M. M., Dodge, K. A., Shaw, D. S., Pettit, G. S., & Bates, J. E. (2009). Trajectories of physical discipline: Early childhood antecedents and developmental outcomes. *Child Development, 80,* 1385–1402.

42. Berlin, L. J., Ipsa, J. M., Fine, M. A., Malone, P. S., Brooks-Gunn, J., Brady-Smith, C., et al. (2009). Correlates and consequences of spanking and verbal punishment for low-income white, African-American, and Mexican-American toddlers. *Child Development, 80,* 1403–1420; Erath, S. A., Bierman, K. L., & the Conduct Problems Prevention Research Group. (2006). Aggressive marital conflict, maternal harsh punishment, and child aggressive-disruptive behavior: Evidence for direct and mediate relations. *Journal of Family Psychology, 20,* 217–226; Taylor, C. A., Manganello, J. A., Lee, S. J., & Rice, J. C. (2010). Mothers' spanking of 3-year-old children and subsequent risk of children's aggressive behavior. *Pediatrics, 125,* e1057–e1065.

43. For a comprehensive review of these interventions, and the research base supporting them, see Roberts, M. W. (2008). Parent training. In M. Hersen & A. M. Gross (Eds.). *Handbook of clinical Psychology,* Volume 2: *Children and adolescents* (pp. 653–693). Hoboken, NJ: John Wiley & Sons.

44. See, for example, Hembree-Kigin, T. L. & McNeil, C. B. (1995). *Parent-child interaction therapy.* New York: Plenum Press; McMahon, R. J. & Forehand, R. L. (2003). *Helping the noncompliant child* (2nd ed.). New York: Guilford Press.

45. Kochanska, G., Forman, D. R., Aksan, N., & Dunbar, S. B. (2005). Pathways to conscience: Early mother-child mutually responsive orientation and children's moral emotion, conduct, and cognition. *Journal of Child Psychology and Psychiatry, 46,* 19–34; Kochanska, G., Barry, R. A., Aksan, N., & Boldt, L. J. (2008). A developmental model of maternal and child contributions to disruptive conduct: The first six years. *Journal of Child Psychology and Psychiatry, 49,* 1220–1227.

46. Roberts, Parent training.

47. Ladd, G. W., LeSieur, K., & Profilet, S. M. (1993). Direct parental influences on young children's peer relations. In S. Duck (Ed.), *Learning about relationships* (Vol. 2, pp. 152–183). London: Sage; Laird, R. D., Pettit, G. S., Mize, J., & Lindsey, E. (1994). Mother–child conversations about peers: Contributions to competence. *Family Relations, 43,* 425–432; Mize, J., & Pettit, G. S. (1997). Mothers' social

coaching, mother–child relationship style, and children's peer competence: Is the medium the message? *Child Development, 68,* 312–332.

48. Russell, A., Pettit, G. S., & Mize, J. (1998). Horizontal qualities in parent–child relationships: Parallels with and possible consequences for children's peer relationships, *Developmental Review, 18,* 313–352; Lindsey, E. W., & Mize, J. (2000). Parent–child physical and pretense play: Links to children's social competence. *Merrill-Palmer Quarterly, 46,* 1479–1498; Pettit, G. S., Brown, E. G., Mize, J., & Lindsey, E. (1998). Mothers' and fathers' socializing behaviors in three contexts: Links with children's peer competence. *Merrill-Palmer Quarterly, 44,* 385–394.

49. Mounts, N. S., & Steinberg, L. (1995). An ecological analysis of peer influence on adolescent grade point average and drug use. *Developmental Psychology, 31,* 915–922.

50. Furman, W., Simon, V. A., Shaffer, L., & Bouchey, H. A. (2002). Adolescents' working models and styles for relationships with parents, friends, and romantic partners. *Child Development, 73,* 241–255.

51. Fletcher, A. C., Darling, N. E., Steinberg, L., & Dornbusch, S. M. (1995). The company they keep: Relation of adolescents' adjustment and behavior to their friends' perceptions of authoritative parenting in the social network. *Developmental Psychology, 31,* 300–310; Mason, C. A., Cauce, A. M., Gonzales, N., & Hiraga, Y. (1996). Neither too sweet nor too sour: Problem peers, maternal control, and problem behavior in African American adolescents. *Child Development, 67,* 2115–2130.

52. Sim, T. N. (2000). Adolescent psychosocial competence: The importance and role of regard for parents. *Journal of Research on Adolescence, 10,* 49–64.

53. Fuligni, A. J., & Eccles, J. S. (1993). Perceived parent–child relationships and early adolescents' orientation toward peers. *Developmental Psychology, 29,* 622–632.

54. Hoeve, M., Dubas, J. S., Eichelsheim, V. I., van der Laan, P. H., Smeenk, W., & Gerris, J.R.M. (2009). The relationship between parenting and delinquency: A meta-analysis. *Journal of Abnormal Child Psychology, 37,* 749–775; Laird, R. D., Criss, M. M., Pettit, G. S., Dodge, K. A., & Bates, J. E. (2008). Parents' monitoring knowledge attenuates the link between antisocial friends and adolescent delinquent behavior. *Journal of Abnormal Child Psychology, 36,* 299–310; McCoy, S. I., Jewell, N. P., Hubbard, A., Gerdts, C. E., Doherty, I. A., Padian, N. S., & Minnis, A. M. (2010). A trajectory analysis of alcohol and marijuana use among Latino adolescents in San Francisco, California. *Journal of Adolescent Health, 47,* 564–574.

55. See Crouter, A. C., & Head, M. R. (2002). Parental monitoring and knowledge of children. In M. H. Bornstein (Ed.), *Handbook of parenting*: Vol. 3. *Being and becoming a parent* (2nd ed., pp. 461–483). Mahwah, NJ: Erlbaum.

56. Dick, D., Latendresse, S. J., Lansford, J. E., Budde, J. P., Goate, A., Dodge, K. A., . . . Bates, J. E. (2009). Role of GABRA2 in trajectories of externalizing behavior across development and evidence of moderation by parental monitoring. *Archives of General Psychiatry, 66,* 649–658.

57. Véronneau, M. & Dishion, T. J. (2010). Predicting change in early adolescent problem behavior in the middle school years: A mesosystemic perspective on parenting and peer experiences. *Journal of Abnormal Child Psychology, 38,* 1125–1137.

58. See, for example, Dishion, T. J., Nelson, S. E., & Kavanagh, K. (2003). The family check-up with high-risk young adolescents: preventing early onset substance use by parent monitoring. *Behavior Therapy, 34,* 553–571; Schinke, S. P., Fang, L., & Cole, K. C. (2009). Computer-delivered parent involvement intervention to prevent substance use among adolescent girls. *Preventive Medicine, 49,* 429–435.

59. Gottman, J. & DeClaire, J. (1997). *Raising an emotionally intelligent child.* New York: Fireside, p. 21.

60. Ibid., 24.

61. Ibid.; Ramsden, S. R., & Hubbard, J. A. (2002). Family expressiveness and parental emotion coaching: Their role in children's emotion regulation and aggression; Shortt, J. W., Stoolmiller, M., Smith-Shine, J. N., Eddy, J. M., & Sheeber, L. (2010). Maternal emotion coaching, adolescent anger regulation, and siblings' externalizing symptoms. *Journal of Child Psychology and Psychiatry, 51,* 799–808.

62. Gottman, J., Katz, L., & Hooven, C. (1996). *Meta-emotion: How families communicate emotionally, links to child peer relations and other developmental outcomes.* Mahwah, NJ: Lawrence Erlbaum.

63. Katz, L. F., & Windecker-Nelsen, B. (2006). Domestic violence, emotion coaching, and child aggression. *Journal of Family Psychology, 20,* 56–67.

64. Havinghurst, S. S., Wilson, K. R., Harley, A. E., Prior, M. R., & Kehoe, C. (2010). Tuning in to kids: Improving socialization practices in parents of preschool children—findings from a community trial. *Journal of Child Psychology and Psychiatry, 51,* 1342–1350.

65. Connell, A. M., & Goodman, S. H. (2002). The association between psychopathology in fathers versus mothers and children's internalizing and externalizing behavior problems: A meta-analysis. *Psychological Bulletin, 128,* 746–773.

66. See, for example, Goodman, S. H., & Gottlib, J. H. (1999). Risk for psychopathology in the children of depressed mothers: A developmental model for understanding mechanisms of transmission. *Psychological Review, 106,* 458–490.

67. Garber, J., Ciesla, J. A., McCauley, E., & Diamond, G. (2011). Remission of depression in parents: Links to health functioning in their children. *Child Development, 82,* 226–243.

68. Riley, A. W., Valdez, C. R., Barrueco, S., Mills, C., Beardslee, W., Sandler, I., & Rawal, P. (2008). Development of a family-based program to reduce risk and promote resilience among families affected by maternal depression: Theoretical basis and program description. *Clinical Child and Family Psychology Review, 11,* 12–29.

69. Valdez, C. R., Mills, C. L., Barrueco, S., Leis, J., & Riley, A. (2011). A pilot study of a family-focused intervention for children and families affected by maternal depression. *Journal of Family Therapy, 33,* 3–19.

70. Hetherington, E. M., & Stanley-Hagan, M. (2002). Parenting in divorced and remarried families. In M. H. Bornstein (Ed.), *Handbook of parenting*: Vol. 3. *Being and becoming a parent* (2nd ed., pp. 287–315). Mahwah, NJ: Erlbaum; Federal Interagency Forum on Child and Family Statistics. (2009). *America's children: Key national indicators of well-being, 2009.* Washington, DC: U.S. Government Printing Office.

71. Amato, P. R. (2001). Children of divorce in the 1990s: An update of the Amato and Keith (1991) meta-analysis. *Journal of Family Psychology, 15,* 355–370; Wolfinger, N. H. (2000). Beyond the intergenerational transmission of divorce: Do people replicate the patterns of marital instability they grew up with? *Journal of Family Issues, 21,* 1061–1086.

72. Amato, Children of divorce in the 1990s; Kunz, J. (2001). Parental divorce and children's interpersonal relationships: A meta-analysis. *Journal of Divorce and Remarriage, 34,* 19–47; Reifman, A., Villa, L. C., Amans, J. A., Rethinam, V., & Telesca, T. Y. (2001). Children of divorce in the 1990s: A meta-analysis. *Journal of Divorce & Remarriage, 36,* 27–36.

73. Forgatch, M. S., & DeGarmo, D. S. (1999). Parenting through change: An effective prevention program for single mothers. *Journal of Consulting and Clinical Psychology, 67*, 711–724.

74. Wolchik, S. A., Sandler, I. N., Millsap, R. E., Plummer, B. A., Greene, S. M., Anderson, E. R., . . . Haine, R. A. (2003). Six-year follow-up of preventive interventions for children of divorce: A randomized controlled trial. *Journal of the American Medical Association, 288*, 1874–1881.

CHAPTER 10

1. Sparks and Duncan, this volume (chapter 5).

2. Hirschi, T. (2004). Self-control and crime. In R. F. Baumeister & K. D. Vohs (Eds.), *Handbook of self-regulation: Research, theory and applications.* New York: Guilford Press; Gottfredson, M. R., & Hirschi, T. (1990). *A general theory of crime.* Stanford, CA: Stanford University Press.

3. Tremblay, R. E., Hartup, W. W., & Archer, J. (Eds.). (2005). *Developmental origins of aggression.* New York: The Guilford Press.

4. http://www.pnas.org/cgi/doi/10.1073/pnas.1010076108i8

5. Shanker, S., Casenhiser, D., & Stieben, J. (2011). *Understanding the nature of self-regulation.* Manuscript submitted for publication.

6. http://www.environmentalhealth.ca/fall08brain.html

7. Field, T. (2007). *The amazing infant.* New York: Wiley-Blackwell.

8. http://www.mflmarmac.k12.ia.us/School%20Website/high_school/student_gallery/writing/family_decline.htm

9. Hirsch-Pasek, K., Golinkoff, M., Berk, L., & Singer, D. (2008). *A mandate for playful learning in preschool: Applying the scientific evidence.* New York: Oxford University Press.

10. Louv, R. (2005). *Last child in the woods.* New York: Algonquin Books.

11. Ratey, J. R. (2008). *Spark: The revolutionary new science of exercise and the brain.* New York: Little, Brown & Co.

12. Staples, A. D. & Bates, J. E. (in press). Children's sleep deficits and cognitive and behavioral adjustment. In M. El-Sheikh (Ed.), *Sleep and development: Familial and socio-cultural considerations.*

13. Shanker, S. (in press). Emotion regulation through the ages. In A. Foolen, U. Luedke, J. Zlatev, & T. Racine (Eds.), *Moving ourselves, moving others: The role of (e)motion in intersubjectivity, consciousness and language.* London: John Benjamins.

14. Mischel, W., Shoda, Y., & Rodriguez, M. L. (1989). Delay of gratification in children. *Science, 244*, 933–938.

15. Lewis, M. D., Granic, I., Lamm, C., Zelazo, P. D., Stieben, J., Todd, R. M., . . . Pepler, D. (2008). Changes in the neural bases of emotion regulation associated with clinical improvement in children with behavior problems. *Development and Psychopathology, 20*(03), 913–939.

16. Robinson, C., Mandleco, B., Olsen, S. F., & Hart, C. H. (1995). Authoritative, authoritarian, and permissive parenting practices: Development of a new measure. *Psychological Reports, 77*, 819–830.

17. O'Keefe, M. (2005, April). *Teen dating violence: A review of risk factors and prevention efforts.* Harrisburg, PA: VAWnet, a project of the National Resource Center

on Domestic Violence/Pennsylvania Coalition Against Domestic Violence. Retrieved from: http://www.vawnet.org

18. Mahler, M., Pine, F., & Bergman, A. (1973). *The Psychological Birth of the Human Infant*. New York: Basic Books.

19. Bradley, S. (2000). *Affect regulation and the development of psychopathology*. New York: Guilford Press.

20. Cloninger, C. R. (1987). Neurogenetic adaptive mechanisms in alcoholism. *Science, 236,* 410–416.

21. Schore, A. (1994). *Affect regulation and the origin of the self.* New York: Psychology Press.

22. Greenspan, S. I. (1979). Intelligence and adaptation: an integration of psychoanalytic and *Piagetian developmental psychology*. New York: International Universities Press; Greenspan, S. I., & Greenspan, N. T. (1981). *The Clinical interview of the child*. New York: McGraw-Hill; Greenspan, S. I. (1989). The development of the ego: implications for personality theory, psychopathology, and the psychotherapeutic process. Madison, CT: International Universities Press; Greenspan, S. I. (1997). *Developmentally based psychotherapy*. Madison, CT: International Universities Press.

23. Schunk, D. H., & Ertmer, P. A. (2000). Self-regulation and academic learning: self-efficacy enhancing interventions. In M. Boekaerts, P. R. Pintrich, & M. Zeidner (Eds.), *Handbook of self-regulation* (pp. 631–649). San Diego: Academic Press.

24. Campos, J. J., Mumme, D. L., Kermoian, R., & Campos, R. G. (1994). A functionalist perspective on the nature of emotion (pp. 284–303). *Monographs of the Society for Research in Child Development, 59*(2–3, Serial No. 240).

25. Greenspan, The development of the ego.

26. Panksepp, J. (1998). *Affective neuroscience: the foundations of human and animal emotions*. New York: Oxford University Press.

27. Greenspan, S. I. (1997). *The growth of the mind and the endangered origins of intelligence*. Reading, MA: Addison-Wesley.

28. Greenspan, S., & Shanker, S. *The first idea: How symbols, language and intelligence evolved from our primate ancestors to modern humans*. Jackson, TN: Da Capo Press, Perseus Books, 2004.

29. Porges, S. (2011). *The polyvagal theory: Neurophysiological foundations of emotions, attachment, communication and self-regulation*. New York: W.W. Norton.

30. Duhn, L. (2010). The importance of touch in the development of attachment. *Advances in Neonatal Care*, (10), 294–300.

31. Wenar, C. (1982). On negativism. *Human Development, 2,* 1–23.

32. Bradley, *Affect regulation*.

33. Zajonc, R. B. (1998). Emotions. In D. T. Gilbert, S. T. Fiske & G. Lindzey (Eds.), *The handbook of social psychology* (4th ed., Vol. 2, pp. 591–632). Boston: McGraw-Hill.

34. Goodenough, F. L. (1931). *Anger in young children*. Institute for Child Welfare Monographs. Minneapolis: University of Minnesota Press.

35. Greenspan, S. I. & Lewis, N. B. (2000). *Building healthy minds*. Cambridge, MA: Da Capo/Perseus Books.

36. Central to the developmental individualized relationship-based (DIR) model of intervention developed by Stanley Greenspan and Serena Wieder is the importance of mobilizing a child's natural interests, which, as Bruner argued, is

essential for the learning interactions that enable the different parts of the mind and brain to work together and to build successively higher levels of social, emotional, and intellectual capacities. According to this model, it is absolutely critical that clinicians, parents, and teachers follow the child's natural emotional interests and at the same time challenge the child toward greater and greater mastery of his social, emotional, and intellectual capacities. But the immediate goals are to encourage the child's initiative and purposeful behavior, deepen his engagement, enhance his capacity to initiate joint attention, and develop his communicative capacities, always following the child's lead.

37. Casenhiser, D., Shanker, S., & Stieben, J. (in press). Learning through interaction. *Autism*.

38. http://www.parl.gc.ca/Content/SEN/Committee/392/soci/rep/rep 08feb08-e.pdf

39. kidshavestresstoo.php

40. Gordon, M. (2007). *Roots of empathy: Changing the world child by child*. Markham, ON: Thomas Allen Publishers.

41. Diamond, A., Barnett, W. S., Thomas, J., & Munro, S. (2007, November 30). Preschool program improves cognitive control. *Science 318*, 1387–1388 + 24 pp. Supplemental Online Material. Retrieved from http://www.sciencemag.org/cgi/content/full/317/5838/1387/DC1

42. Louv, *Last child in the woods*; Ratey, *Spark*.

About the Editors
and Contributors

EDITORS

SHARNA OLFMAN is a professor of clinical and developmental psychology at Point Park University and a clinical psychologist in private practice. She is the editor/author of the Childhood in America book series for Praeger/ABC-CLIO. Her books include *The Sexualization of Childhood* (2008), *Bipolar Children* (2007), *No Child Left Different* (2006), *Child Honoring* (coedited with Raffi Cavoukian, 2006), *Childhood Lost* (2005), and *All Work and No Play* (2003). Dr. Olfman is a member of the Council of Human Development and a partner in the Alliance for Childhood. She has written and lectured internationally on the subjects of children's mental health and parenting. She was the founder and director of the annual Childhood and Society Symposium, a multidisciplinary think tank on childhood advocacy from 2001 to 2008.

BRENT DEAN ROBBINS is an associate professor of psychology and director of the Psychology Program at Point Park University. He is editor-in-chief of *Janus Head: Journal of Interdisciplinary Studies in Literature, Continental Philosophy, and Phenomenological Psychology,* and a recipient of the American Psychological Association's Harmi Carari Early Career Award. Dr. Robbins is member-at-large and conference coordinator for Division 32 of the American Psychological Association, and also editor of the Division's blog. His published research has included mixed-method investigations of emotion, embodiment, and the medicalization of the body in contemporary Western culture, with particular attention to the implications of these findings for the treatment of mental illness.

CONTRIBUTORS

LAURA E. BERK is distinguished professor of psychology emerita at Illinois State University. She has published widely in the fields of early childhood development and education, focusing on the effects of school environments on children's development, the social origins and functional significance of children's private speech, and the role of make-believe play in the development of self-regulation. Her book for parents and teachers is *Awakening Children's Minds: How Parents and Teachers Can Make a Difference*, and she is coauthor of *Private Speech: From Social Interaction to Self-Regulation, Scaffolding Children's Learning: Vygotsky and Early Childhood Education*, and *A Mandate for Playful Learning in Preschool*. She is the author of three textbooks in child and human development: *Child Development*; *Infants, Children, and Adolescents*; and *Development Through the Lifespan*.

BARRY L. DUNCAN is director of the Heart and Soul of Change Project (http://www.heartandsoulofchange.com) and author or coauthor of 15 books, including *On Becoming a Better Therapist* and *The Heart and Soul of Change*. Dr. Duncan codeveloped the Partners for Change Outcome Management System to give clients the voice they deserve and provide feedback about the clients' response to services, thus enabling more effective care tailored to client preferences. He can be reached at barrylduncan@comcast.net.

JIM GOTTSTEIN graduated from Harvard Law School in 1978 and lives in Anchorage, Alaska. Since 2002, he has devoted the bulk of his time pro bono to the Law Project for Psychiatric Rights (PsychRights)—which he cofounded—whose mission is to mount a strategic litigation campaign against forced psychiatric drugging and electroshock across the United States. In June 2006, Mr. Gottstein won a landmark decision in the Alaska Supreme Court: *Myers v. Alaska Psychiatric Institute*, which ruled Alaska's forced drugging procedures unconstitutional. *Myers* has been called "the most important State Supreme Court decision" on forced drugging in 20 years. He has won three other important Alaska Supreme Court decisions since then, which are described on the PyschRights website. Mr. Gottstein is most known around the

United States and internationally for subpoenaing and releasing the *Zyprexa Papers* in late 2006, resulting in a series of *New York Times* articles and an editorial calling for a Congressional investigation. In January 2009, Eli Lilly pled guilty and agreed to pay $1.4 billion in civil and criminal fines for the activities revealed by the *Zyprexa Papers*. He has also devoted considerable time trying to make alternatives to psychiatric drugs available in Alaska through Soteria-Alaska, CHOICES Inc., and Peer Properties. Mr. Gottstein serves on the board of directors of the National Association for Rights and Advocacy (NARPA) and the International Society for Ethical Psychology and Psychiatry.

ADENA B. MEYERS is an associate professor of psychology and member of the School of Psychology Graduate Program Faculty at Illinois State University. She received her doctorate in clinical-community psychology from the University of Illinois at Urbana-Champaign and is a licensed clinical psychologist. She is interested in contextual influences on child and adolescent development, with an emphasis on family-, school-, and community-based interventions designed to promote children's social and emotional functioning. Her publications have focused on school-based consultation as well as adolescent pregnancy, parenthood, and sexual development. She has served as a consultant to the Collaborative for Academic, Social, and Emotional Learning (CASEL), and her current work involves evaluation research related to school-based preventive interventions.

GWEN OLSEN spent more than a decade as a sales representative in the pharmaceutical industry working for health care giants such as Johnson & Johnson, Bristol-Myers Squibb, and Abbott Laboratories. A well-known media resource, she has been in numerous print, radio, and television media reports, and she has testified before Congress and the FDA. A 2007 Human Rights Award winner, she currently devotes her time to writing, speaking engagements, and health activism. She is the author of the award-winning book *Confessions of an Rx Drug Pusher.*

STUART SHANKER is distinguished research professor of philosophy and psychology at York University and director of the Milton and Ethel Harris Research Initiative at York University. He is the recipient of a $7 million grant from the Harris Steel Foundation to establish MEHRI, a state-of-the-art cognitive and social neuroscience center. Among his monographs are *Apes, Language and the Human Mind* (with Sue Savage-Rumbaugh and Talbot Taylor, 1998); *Wittgenstein's Remarks on the Foundations of AI* (1998); *Toward a Psychology of Global Interdependency* (with Stanley Greenspan, 2002); *The First Idea* (with Stanley Greenspan, 2004); *Early Years Study II* (with J. Fraser Mustard and Margaret McCain, 2007); and *El Rizoma de la Racionalidad* (with Pedro Reygadas, 2008). He is the editor of several collections, among them *The Routledge History of Philosophy* (with G.H.R. Parkinson, 1994–2000); *Language, Culture, Self* (with David Bakhurst, 2001); *Ludwig Wittgenstein: Critical Assessments* (with David Kilfoyle, 2002); *Psychodynamic Diagnostic Manual* (a member of the PDM Steering Committee, 2006); and *Human Development in the 21st Century* (with Alan Fogel and Barbara King, 2008). Dr. Shanker has just been appointed the director of EPIC, an international initiative created to promote the educational potential in children by enhancing their self-regulation. He has served as the director of the Council of Human Development for the past 10 years and the director of the Canada-Cuba Research Alliance for the past six years, and he was the first president of the Council of Early Child Development in Canada. Over the past decade, he has served as an advisor on early child development to government organizations across Canada and the United States and countries around the world.

JACQUELINE A. SPARKS is associate professor in the Couple and Family Therapy Program, Department of Human Development and Family Studies, University of Rhode Island. Her interests include using client feedback protocols in clinical training, feedback and outcome in couple and family therapy, transforming systems of care to privilege client goals and promote social justice, and critical analysis of child psychotropic prescription. She is coauthor of *Heroic Client* and *Heroic Clients, Heroic Agencies: Partners for Change;* cofounder of the Heroicagencies Listserv; leader, Heart and Soul of Change Project; scientific advisory board member, Mindfreedom International; and board member, International Society for Ethical Psychology and Psychiatry.

TONY STANTON is an adult and child psychiatrist who has devoted the greater part of his career to directing and consulting with community mental health programs for adults, children, and adolescents. These have included inpatient and outpatient facilities, residential programs, and programs for the developmentally disabled and learning disabled. For the past 21 years, he has divided his work between Washington State and California. He completed his training in child psychiatry at Langley Porter Neuropsychiatric Institute (UCSF) where he continued to serve as a member of the clinical staff (supervising residents and fellows in child psychiatry) until he moved to Washington State. He is board certified in adult and child psychiatry.

GEORGE STONE holds an MA in anthropology (Arizona '72) and an MSW (University of Maryland at Baltimore '80). He studied privately with Milton H. Erickson, MD; Gregory Bateson; Jay Haley; Cloe Madanes; and Braulio Montalvo. He has 39 years of experience as a therapist, supervisor, and teacher. His work synthesizes the strategic family therapy of Jay Haley and Cloe Madanes with the symbolic anthropology of Victor and Edith Turner. Mr. Stone has dedicated his career to helping families solve their own problems without the use of psychiatric medication or hospitalization.

ROBERT WHITAKER is the author of *Mad in America*, a history of the treatment of the mentally ill in the United States, and *Anatomy of an Epidemic: Magic Bullets, Psychiatric Drugs, and the Astonishing Rise of Mental Illness in America*. His newspaper and magazine articles on mental illness and the pharmaceutical industry have garnered several national awards, including a George Polk Award for medical writing and a National Association of Science Writers Award for best magazine article. *Anatomy of an Epidemic* won a 2010 award for best investigative journalism, book category, from the Investigative Reporters and Editors organization.

Index